Diabetes

A Guide to Living Well

Gary Arsham, MD, PhD & Ernest Lowe

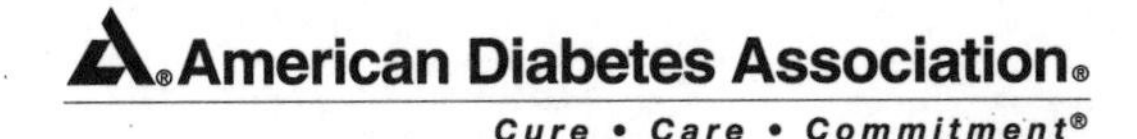

Director, Book Publishing, John Fedor; *Associate Director, Consumer Books,* Sherrye Landrum; *Editor,* Laurie Guffey; *Associate Director, Book Production,* Peggy M. Rote; *Composition,* Circle Graphics, Inc.; *Cover Design,* Koncept Inc.; *Printer,* Port City Press.

Printed in the United States of America
1 3 5 7 9 10 8 6 4 2

The suggestions and information contained in this publication are generally consistent with the *Clinical Practice Recommendations* and other policies of the American Diabetes Association, but they do not represent the policy or position of the Association or any of its boards or committees. Reasonable steps have been taken to ensure the accuracy of the information presented. However, the American Diabetes Association cannot ensure the safety or efficacy of any product or service described in this publication. Individuals are advised to consult a physician or other appropriate health care professional before undertaking any diet or exercise program or taking any medication referred to in this publication. Professionals must use and apply their own professional judgment, experience, and training and should not rely solely on the information contained in this publication before prescribing any diet, exercise, or medication. The American Diabetes Association—its officers, directors, employees, volunteers, and members—and the authors assume no responsibility or liability for personal or other injury, loss, or damage that may result from the suggestions or information in this publication.

∞ The paper in this publication meets the requirements of the ANSI Standard Z39.48-1992 (permanence of paper).

ADA titles may be purchased for business or promotional use or for special sales. To purchase this book in large quantities, or for custom editions of this book with your logo, contact Lee Romano Sequeira, Special Sales & Promotions, at the address below, or at LRomano@diabetes.org or 703-299-2046.

American Diabetes Association
1701 North Beauregard Street
Alexandria, Virginia 22311

Library of Congress Cataloging-in-Publication Data

Lowe, Ernest.
Diabetes : a guide to living well / Ernest Lowe & Gary Arsham.—4th ed.
p. cm.
Includes index.
ISBN 1-58040-209-7 (pbk. : alk. paper)
1. Diabetes—Popular works. I. Arsham, Gary M. II. Title.

RC660.4.L69 2004
616.4'62—dc22 2004047721

Dedication

To Diana Silver Arsham and Grace O'Reilly Lowe, who could easily write a sequel to this book called *Diabetics: A Guide to Living Well with Them.*

To my parents, Florence and Sanford Arsham, and my physician while growing up, Max Miller, who gave me the guidance and freedom to live well.

—Gary

To John Menscher and Michael Barricks, whose skilled laser treatment enabled me to keep 20/20 vision.

—Ernest

Contents

PART FOUR
Women and Children Living Well

Acknowledgments

Many people have made valuable contributions to *Diabetes: A Guide to Living Well*—fellow people with diabetes (patients and friends) as well as professional colleagues.

We wish to thank Everett Ai, Carol Alston, Robert Barnes, Peter Barrett, Patrick Bean, Ken Burke, Philip R. Calanchini, Larry Catus, Cathy Corum, Leona Dang, Wayne Davis, Joan Enns, Fran Fernandez, Betty Fukuyama, Diana Guthrie, Dwight Holing, Peggy Huang, Larry Hulbert, Chris Kilduff, Barry S. Levin, Maureen McGrath, Nancy Key Nelson, Fran Nereu, Jan Norman, Linda Parker, Sheila Perez, Donna Radcliffe, Vicky Sears, the late Nanci Stern, Wendy Ullman, Helen Wall, Ben and Bonnie Weyhing, Seena Wolf, patients of the Early Treatment Diabetic Retinopathy Study, and the many others who supported our work with their knowledge and experience.

Special thanks go to George Cleveland and also Caroline Danielson, our editor for the first edition, for helping to bring this book to completion. We are grateful to Donna Hoel and David Wexler for their assistance and guidance with the second edition. We appreciate the help of Jeff Braun with the third edition. We are especially appreciative of the writing and editorial work done on the third edition by Grace Lowe, Ernie's wife. We thank our friend and colleague, Cathy Feste, for her help in writing the sections on women and children. We couldn't have done it without you! Thanks to Sherrye Landrum and Laurie Guffey for their commitment to and work on this fourth edition.

Preface

We wrote *Diabetes: A Guide to Living Well* so you can learn to truly live well with diabetes. It is possible, and we can show you how. In this book we tell you about two different levels of diabetes management, moderate control and best control, and help you choose the best one for you now. This book will show you how to succeed in diabetes wellness as you work your way toward the best level of control.

The Living Well approach is based on our lives with diabetes. We know diabetes personally and professionally. Your writing team has logged over 135 years of living with diabetes! We have first-hand knowledge of the challenges, threats, and gifts—yes, gifts—of diabetes.

The goal of diabetes management is to keep your blood sugar, cholesterol, and blood pressure levels where they should be so you feel well and avoid complications, particularly heart disease and stroke. If you think of that goal as the seat of a four-legged chair, the legs supporting it are eating well, being physically active, taking any pills or insulin, and managing stress.

When any leg isn't working properly, the whole chair is unstable. When you pay attention to all four legs, your chair is steady.

Throughout the book, we encourage you to pay attention to all four legs.

This book helps you balance taking care of your diabetes with the other demands in your life, and helps you choose the program you can stick with today.

You may have much to learn, many skills to gain, and some habits to change as you work on living well, especially if you are new to diabetes. Throughout this book, you'll find ideas for making this process of learning and changing easier to handle. You'll also find many techniques for increasing your willingness to take better care of yourself.

Diabetes is a condition requiring a balance between your own day-to-day decision-making and your doctor's guidance on diabetes health issues. We include detailed information on two Living Well Programs so you can decide how you want to successfully manage your diabetes right now. But work with your doctor and diabetes care team as you decide exactly how to handle pill or insulin dose; the balance between food, insulin or pills, and physical activity; or treatment of acute problems like hypoglycemia or infections. In no way do we encourage you to make these fundamental medical decisions completely on your own. And keep working toward best control, in order to enjoy the best possible health.

In writing this book, we have deepened our own capacity for living well with diabetes. We hope reading it helps you do the same.

Gary Arsham, MD, PhD
Ernest Lowe

Introduction

This book is about options and personal choices. We can choose how to live with diabetes. We can't decide not to have it, but we can decide to live a full and satisfying life, rejecting all images of ourselves as ill or disabled. No matter what our physical condition, we can choose to live well. The act of choosing becomes the foundation of our ability to manage diabetes effectively.

Nobody asked me if I wanted to have diabetes. I just started feeling lousy, losing weight, and getting thirsty. And there I was—diabetic. I thought my life was ruined. But then I said, "No, dammit! This may not go away, but I'm going to call the shots. My life is more than a defective pancreas."

Living well depends less on how we care for our diabetes than on how we care for ourselves. Each of us has a pattern of living that includes our individual needs, style, abilities, and physical characteristics. The wellness plan we choose will work only if it fits this pattern. We can't make decisions about diabetes care as if diabetes is the only thing we have to consider in life.

> The anger, frustration, and all of those feelings aren't going to take the diabetes away. You have to find a level ground and decide, "Okay, this is the way I am now and I'd better learn what I'm supposed to do and what I'm not supposed to do and live with it, because that's the way it's going to be."
>
> **—Norma, 58**

So choose the Living Well program that will work best for you. Read this book in whatever order feels right to you. Work on the subjects that interest you the most. Find the plan that you can follow comfortably now. Work to find a healthy balance between quality of life and care of your diabetes. And keep working to improve your diabetes care until you have achieved what we call "best," optimal, or tight control, found in the intensive program.

The Living Well Programs will ask you to work toward the following goals.

- Improve your blood sugar control and continue improving it to the best level you can.
- Follow a meal plan that is moderate and healthy (Chapter 8).
- Lose weight if you are overweight.
- Engage in physical activity regularly (Chapter 9).
- Know how to prevent and treat low blood sugar (Chapter 10).
- Work to increase your willingness to be healthy (Chapters 2–3).
- Develop support networks (Chapter 13).
- Learn to handle stress well (Chapter 12).
- Keep your cholesterol and blood pressure levels in a healthy range (by losing weight, eating right, exercising a little most days, and managing stress).
- Get the amount of rest and sleep you need.
- Know the warning signs for complications (Chapter 11).

As you work to achieve these goals, if you select the Moderate Program instead of the Intensive Program, you may feel guilt, anxiety, or conflict about making a "bad" choice. Bring these feelings out into the open and look at them. You need to accept your decision about your level of care without self-blame. Read about the different programs and understand the risks and benefits of different care options. Make an informed decision, then accept your decision. You can always keep working on your diabetes goals as you move toward the best control.

Living well with diabetes is easier if you stay flexible and are willing to keep learning about the rapid changes in diabetes management. There are new skills to be learned, and behaviors will need changing as you gain new information. We have included hints and strategies in this book to make that learning process easier.

Throughout this book we offer advice on how you can motivate yourself to live well. It's hard to change habits, and all of us feel resistant and rebellious at times. That's odd when we are the ones who will benefit from the changes. You may have to spend time learning more about yourself and how you are reacting to having diabetes, about how you really think and feel about your condition. To take advantage of improvements in diabetes care, you may need to pay attention to the feelings, beliefs, and patterns of behavior that sometimes hold you back.

Living well requires accepting uncertainty and staying motivated despite this uncertainty. We want to feel that what we do to take care of ourselves will actually work. Research shows that for most of us, good blood sugar control means we can avoid serious complications of diabetes. If you already have complications, good control helps slow down and sometimes reverse the damage.

Clearly, managing diabetes is a matter of balance—doing your best to live a rewarding life, without dwelling on possible problems in the future. One way of neutralizing uncertainty about the future is to make the present rewarding. Learn to accept each moment as a source of benefit, no matter what happens. This way, you're prepared for whatever the future brings. Diabetes can teach us how to do this.

Having diabetes is a challenge, a burden, a transformation, and a blessing. So let's accept it as a gracious gift and let it teach us to live our years well.

PART ONE

Learning to Live Well

CHAPTER

1

Life After Diagnosis

If you have recently discovered that you have diabetes, take a deep breath, sigh, and relax for a moment. You are going through a crisis. You may be handling the challenges of this time well, or you may feel overwhelmed by them. In either case, it is a demanding situation, and you need all the breaks you can get.

I really felt sorry for myself when I found out I had diabetes. I still want to know "Why me?" I never did anything to deserve this. Why all of a sudden do I have to stick to a diet and take shots for the rest of my life?

—Carol, 17

Help!

When you have trouble—especially when your health is at stake—a natural response is to become tense and frustrated. When you become tense, it is difficult to find solutions to problems. Begin the process of rescuing yourself by relaxing as deeply as possible, before you begin doing anything else. If you have healthful techniques for relaxing that work for you, use them. Eating, drinking, smoking, watching television, and other common distractions don't count as healthful techniques.

First, Relax

- Begin by saying something like "My only job right now is to relax." For the moment, put all other concerns aside.
- Focus on your breathing, especially the feeling of it as you exhale. You can even sigh as you breathe out if you like. If your mind wanders, gently bring it back to your breath.
- Your body will respond now, if you talk with it. Say, "My right arm is becoming warm and heavy." Repeat this phrase as many times as necessary.
- Now, repeat the phrase for your left arm. "My left arm is becoming warm and heavy." Continue the exercise with your legs.

Within five to ten minutes, your body will translate the feeling of heaviness into relaxation. You can help the process by focusing on the heaviness that develops as you go along, rather than the tensions that remain.

Prayer and meditation can be most effective forms of relaxation. They help you gain insight into the problems you are having. Learn to pay attention to the positive voice inside you guiding you toward better health decisions.

Then, Detach

When difficulties arise, we often feel closed in. We lose perspective and the ability to be creative because we focus on what is wrong. Finding solutions is much easier if we can gain some distance from the difficult situation. This is especially true with serious circumstances, such as being diagnosed with diabetes. No matter how urgent the problem is, you can more effectively solve it if you are calm.

- Adopt a different perspective. Look at your situation from the point of view of an interested, benevolent protector. Say, "Ah, how interesting. Let's look at what we have here. Let's see what we can do about it." Picture yourself as that wise, kind, capable observer.
- Remember a time when things were going well for you, or when you felt very calm and peaceful. See or feel that experience, place, or event. Remember the people that were part of this special time. Let these positive feelings come into the present, reminding you that you are more than someone having a current crisis.
- Think of an area of your life in which you are successful. Appreciate the strengths and skills you demonstrate here. Imagine your success if you act with these qualities on the problem you are now facing.
- Find a humorous point of view for the situation you are in. Laughter is healing and is good for the imagination.
- Let go of any judgments about yourself and your ability to handle problems. Even if you are in total rebellion against the diabetes program, don't condemn yourself. You are acting with power. You just haven't learned to use that power for living well.

First Things First

When you first learn you have diabetes, there are three basic demands to handle:

Practical tasks. You must learn new skills, absorb new information, make decisions you previously did not have to make, and change parts of the way you live.

Emotional tasks. You need to deal with the emotional impact of being told you have a lifelong chronic disease that, as yet, has no cure.

Support tasks. You need to find and use internal and external sources of support.

You may find yourself trying to meet all three needs at the same time, as well as dealing with the other needs in your life. It is very easy to feel overwhelmed in this initial period, so remember that you can't do everything at once. Set priorities with the help of your health care team.

Practical Tasks

The practical demands of diabetes begin long before you feel ready for them. If you have been in the hospital to get your system under control, you know that you cannot be a passive patient. Your life depends on learning a great amount of information very quickly, especially if you have type 1 diabetes. Learning this much at once may make you anxious, since it is hard at first to tell which information is of life-or-death importance. You are still dealing with the emotional shock of the diagnosis and the physical stress of the uncontrolled diabetes, so your mind may not be functioning as clearly as usual.

This is an excellent time to learn a basic lesson of diabetes education: when you don't understand something or when you feel overloaded with information, tell your doctor or diabetes educator Ask for an explanation. Don't just nod your head so the doctor won't think you are stupid. Some health professionals are very good communicators, but others don't notice if you are suffering from information overload.

Sometimes your doctor will be joined by other health professionals. In this case, your basic care will be supervised by a nurse, dietitian, or diabetes educator. Make sure they all speak to you in a way you understand.

Beginning a Treatment Program

Being in charge of your diabetes care may seem to be an enormous responsibility at first, but millions of people with diabetes deal with it and live well every year. Your medical team will provide a lot of support, so you can always get help when you can't figure out what to do. If you consult others with diabetes about simple questions that arise, you can avoid feeling that you are bothering your medical team with too many questions.

Developing excellent patterns of self-care right from the beginning increases your chances of being healthier now and later. You probably already have certain self-care steps you have to do right away, such as take medication or insulin. When you are stable and ready, read Chapter 4 to learn more about the moderate and intensive diabetes care programs. Then choose the one that will work for you now.

See what kind of treatment program your doctor recommends. Then decide if you are in agreement with that advice, and if you are ready to act on it. If you want to maintain tight control but your doctor doesn't support this choice, you may need to find one who does. On the other hand, if your physician urges tight control, but you do not feel ready for it, you can probably negotiate for moderate control. Create a plan for moving in the healthiest direction you can over the next few months.

Learning for Life

Just after diagnosis is probably the most intense period of diabetes learning you will go through. What you learn now will remain with you for years. But living well requires learning for the rest of your life. Diabetes does, too.

You will soon know what a powerful teacher diabetes is, with its many challenges and surprises. You are in the midst of learning the details of care, some of which have life-or-death importance. At this stage, you need to determine which aspects of care are critical.

Diabetes treatment is evolving, so you can expect to continue learning about it for many years. You may learn some of life's important lessons sooner than your friends without diabetes. Our physical condition requires us to accept that we are mortal and encourages us to value the preciousness of life. Many people with diabetes come to see this new appreciation and love for life as a true gift.

To avoid feeling overwhelmed by the amount you have to learn, divide the learning into manageable lessons. Work out a schedule and identify the resources that can assist you. There may be a series of classes at a local hospital or clinic, a diabetes educator (usually a nurse or dietitian) may be available, or your local chapter of the American Diabetes Association (ADA) may offer educational programs and support groups. The members of your health care team have much experience and training in this field, so ask for help as you learn about self care.

Emotional Tasks

Ask a dozen different people how they reacted to being told they have diabetes and you will probably hear a dozen different stories: "It really scared me. My uncle had diabetes and died when he was 40." "No big deal. I don't let things like that get to me." "I was angry for months. I thought it would destroy all of my plans." "I just pulled the covers over my head and felt numb."

The only "right" way to feel is the way you are feeling. In the midst of learning about diabetes management, give yourself time to experience your own emotions. Set aside time to do this. Some people use writing, some take long solitary walks, others pray or meditate. (See the chart below for ways to handle your feelings.)

If you want assistance, remember that it is available, even if you think you are isolated (see Support Tasks, page 10). Try talking to people in your present support network. You also have guaranteed membership in the community of people with diabetes. Or find value in a few sessions with a counselor, psychologist, or social worker.

Look at the chart below. If you are feeling some of the things on the left, try putting some of the ideas on the right into effect.

Feelings	Ideas
You feel helpless or unable to assume your new responsibilities.	It helps to discuss your feelings with other people who have diabetes. They'll reassure you that feelings of being overwhelmed lessen as you begin taking care of yourself.
You feel depressed, fearful, or angry over the many changes in lifestyle that you are expected to make.	Some of these changes are specific to diabetes, but many of them are the basis for healthier living. Regular physical activity and a balanced meal plan are recommended for everyone. It's much easier now for people with diabetes to implement more flexible lifestyle changes, with carbohydrate counting, different medication, multiple daily insulin injections, or the insulin pump.
You are totally depressed about the possibility of developing complications and dying early.	Stories and statistics about diabetes may lead you to believe you are doomed to disability and an early grave. However, recent advances in diabetes care offer you the means of preventing or delaying the onset of any diabetic complications. You are not doomed.

Continued

Feelings	Ideas
You are frustrated about the restrictions you believe diabetes imposes on your life.	Actually, diabetes closes very few doors to you. You are not allowed to fly an airliner or have a job where an insulin reaction would threaten the safety of others. Every other role you seek is open to you.
You are doing everything right, but still feeling extremely anxious.	If you are caught in this pattern, make relaxation and stress management a high priority. Relieving stress lowers your blood glucose and makes you healthier.
You feel unconcerned and insist that diabetes will have no effect on your life. You may even believe that you don't really have the disease.*	Living well with diabetes calls for accepting it as a fact of life—one of major importance. The more you ignore it through little self-care, the greater the impact it can have. If you follow a full wellness program, you will lessen the risks of complications and your body will be healthy enough to benefit from future advances in treatment or a cure.

*Once you get your blood sugar under a moderate degree of control, diabetes has few outward signs. What a "nice" disease it seems to be. The temptation to do little to control it may be strong, especially when you are already getting by with managing the disease. In type 1 diabetes, there is even a "honeymoon period," a few months during which insulin requirements temporarily decrease. However, after this period, they go up again. In type 2, you may do fine for years on pills and then your pancreas "wears out," and you need insulin for better control. Resist the temptation to ignore diabetes!

Support Tasks

Find support right away for dealing with both the practical and emotional issues concerning diabetes. Call on relatives, friends, other people with diabetes, and professionals as soon as you can. You will need comfort, encouragement, and honest feedback on how you are handling things.

Some people are blessed with lots of support networks. Others feel isolated and don't know where to turn. If you feel there is little support available to you, give yourself a chance to be surprised. You may have more resources than you think. Even if you know few people, you are probably no more than two or three phone calls away from dozens of people who are willing to help you cope.

Wherever you live, there are people nearby who are well informed, positive, and helpful. You can contact others through your physician, pharmacist or other health professionals, the ADA, The American Association of Diabetes Educators (AADE), or through people you already know. Let them know you are looking for people who have a positive outlook and who don't mind talking with others about diabetes. If you encounter people who only complain or tell horror stories, cover your ears and stay away from them. You need support, not discouragement. (See Chapter 13 for more on finding support, and Appendix 1 for helpful websites.)

Beginning Well

This questionnaire can help you adjust to diabetes. Use your answers to help you sort out your new priorities. What requests do you need to make of your health care team and support networks? What changes do you need to make in your life to handle this crisis well? Begin with small steps you can easily handle. The most important thing is to get started.

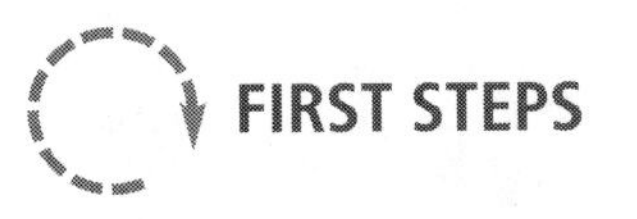

1. Your Support Network

The people I count on for emotional support include:

____

The people who will help me with practical problems, such as getting to an appointment with the doctor or bringing food when I am ill, include:

___

(If you have trouble asking for help) I wouldn't want to ask for help because:

___

How would you answer a friend that gave this reason?

___

(If you feel you need more support) I can increase my support network by:

- ☐ Contacting the American Diabetes Association and The American Association of Diabetes Educators.
- ☐ Joining a support group (either general or specific to diabetes).
- ☐ Joining a computer discussion group.
- ☐ Asking my minister for help.
- ☐ Asking my doctor, diabetes educator, or pharmacist to help me get in touch with other people who have diabetes.
- ☐ Going to a social worker or psychologist.
- ☐ Other___

(If there are people in your life who are discouraging or otherwise negative) I can approach this "anti-support" by:

- ☐ Asking the person involved to change.
- ☐ Changing how I respond.
- ☐ Avoiding the person.
- ☐ Having more contact with people who show a positive attitude.
- ☐ Other___

The strengths I can call on within myself at this time include:

___

A past crisis I handled well was:

____

2. Your Physical Care

☐ I know which parts of diabetes care have life-or-death importance.
☐ I feel satisfied with my physician.
☐ I feel my physician is okay, but I would like him or her to:

____

☐ I feel I need a different doctor because:

____

☐ I feel most certain about the parts of diabetes care I've checked below:

- ☐ Blood glucose monitoring
- ☐ Insulin or medication dosage
- ☐ Low blood sugar
- ☐ Urine testing for ketones
- ☐ Meal planning
- ☐ Exercise or other physical activities
- ☐ The effect of stress on diabetes control
- ☐ The interactions among all of these

(If your budget is limited)
☐ I have located the least expensive source of diabetes supplies.
☐ I have checked the Internet or my support groups for advice.
☐ I have read the ADA's *How to Save up to $3000 a Year on Your Diabetes Costs*.

3. Your Emotional Care

My emotional reactions to the diagnosis of diabetes include the feelings I've checked below.

☐ Anger
☐ Fear
☐ Guilt
☐ Lack of feeling

- ☐ Anxiety
- ☐ Calm
- ☐ Depression
- ☐ Other______________________________

I am dealing with these feelings by:

____

My response to the diagnosis of diabetes includes:

- ☐ I feel overwhelmed by diabetes and find it difficult to handle.
- ☐ I am upset because I have to make too many changes in my life.
- ☐ I feel frightened about what I have heard about complications.
- ☐ I am concerned that diabetes will make it impossible to achieve my life goals.
- ☐ I am worried about doing all the diabetes procedures correctly.
- ☐ I have withdrawn into myself.
- ☐ I don't believe that diabetes is any big deal or that I have to change much.
- ☐ I am dealing with my feelings and with the practical challenges that diabetes has presented.
- ☐ Other______________________________

I can reduce my negative response to diabetes by:

____

4. Your Diabetes Learning Program

- ☐ I have a good idea of what I know and what I still have to learn.
- ☐ I feel confused and need help figuring out what is important to learn.
- ☐ I have enrolled in a diabetes instruction class.
- ☐ I know the members of my health care team and how to contact them.

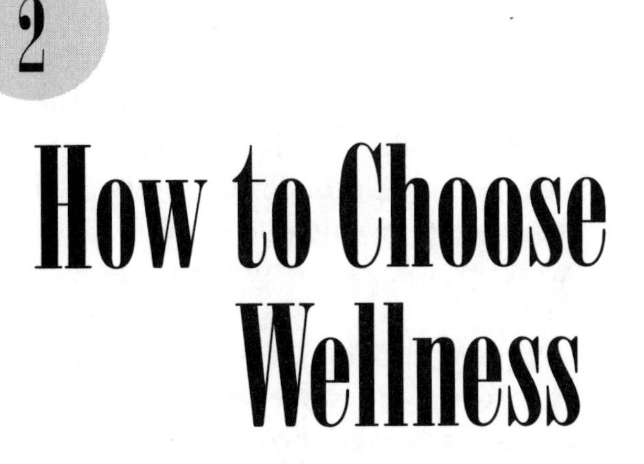

CHAPTER 2

How to Choose Wellness

You are the best available source of support for living well with diabetes. You are always there and you know yourself well. No one else can take care of you as well as you can.

Having diabetes can affect how you feel about yourself, which affects your willingness to live healthfully. The goals of this chapter are to help you:

- become aware of your strengths and resources.
- uncover your beliefs about diabetes.
- learn to neutralize patterns that weaken your ability to care for yourself well.
- handle feelings that come up as you work towards wellness.
- create solutions to your problems that really work.

> For a long time I didn't think I could do it. It seemed like too much work, and I had a lot of other things to worry about. But then I realized I wasn't going to be able to do anything else unless I took better care of myself. And once I started, it got easier and easier.
>
> **—Ron, 45**

You are resourceful. You are stronger, more creative, and more able than you may realize. Some of these strengths can be hidden, or used in only one area of your life. Other strengths can be expressed in negative ways. For example, the teenager who refuses to test or follow a diet and schedule shows great strength of character. Although this strength is focused on rebellion and denial, it is a valuable resource. This teen can learn to turn "won't power" into "will power" and improve his or her self-care.

Or, after months of receiving support, a man still acts as a victim of diabetic complications. He is overwhelmed, helpless, and depressed. Where is his strength now? Perhaps he is strong in the tenacity with which he holds onto his role as victim, refusing to adapt to his situation. Continually feeling sorry for himself takes a great amount of energy. That energy can be harnessed to learn how to live well with diabetes. A negative self-image can be changed to create the flexibility needed to live well with the changes being experienced. Negative feelings can be redirected into positive action.

We often develop skills in one area that we never apply to the rest of our life. Photographers learn about tests, processes, measurements, precision, and combining a complex series of actions to achieve a given result. They have the skills necessary to learn any diabetes wellness program. Salespeople are skilled at communication and persuasion. Perhaps they could use these strengths to sell themselves an improved lifestyle.

Let's explore the resources you can use to live well with diabetes.

Going into Your Storehouse

Do this exercise in a quiet place where you won't be disturbed. At each step, close your eyes and allow both words and images to help you find answers. Make notes before you go to the next step.

1. Think of three areas of your life, large or small, in which you are successful. See yourself in action. What strengths do you demonstrate here?
2. Think of three activities you enjoy. See yourself enjoying them. What personal qualities do you have that allow you to enjoy these activities?
3. What do you believe about yourself that enables you to act with success? With enjoyment?
4. Remember one of the best times in your life. Tell yourself the story of that time or recall scenes from it. Which of your qualities made this such a good time?
5. What strengths do you utilize in your work (or schoolwork, if you are a student)?
6. What strengths do you express in your relationships with friends?
7. What special qualities do you experience only when you are alone?
8. If you were to fulfill your true potential, what hidden qualities would you feel free to express?
9. What qualities would you like to develop?
10. What are some of your most negative traits or limitations?
11. Can you find a strength that each of these limitations contains? Can you think of a way to make them serve you?

Now, review your answers and examine how these qualities can:

- ☐ be your own storehouse for inner strength.
- ☐ help you deal with diabetes.
- ☐ enable you to improve your self-care.
- ☐ help you feel better about your problems.
- ☐ assist when you are fearful or unwilling to do what you know you should do.
- ☐ allow you to resolve problems in relationships with others.

Write down your thoughts or discuss them with a friend.

After you do this exercise, observe your life with these questions in mind. See what traits could help you live well with diabetes. Explore how the qualities you have just identified can improve your self-care.

Recognizing your resources will help you deal with diabetes creatively. You can reinforce this positive step by learning to overcome the negative self-image, limiting beliefs, self-judgments, emotional reactions, and behavioral patterns you experience because of diabetes.

A Case of Mistaken Identity

Beliefs, feelings, and actions create your sense of who you are. You often become closely identified with this sense, forgetting that it is only learned behavior. Many of your limitations seem so real that you can't imagine exceeding them. You forget that you learned to see yourself as inadequate, helpless, rebellious, or sick.

This mistaken identity becomes self-perpetuating. When you believe you are weak and unable to follow a plan, you act weak and unable. You may feel depressed and eat a pint of ice cream, thus making your sugar-clogged body feel uncomfortable. Then you use that feeling as evidence you can't succeed.

In another example, if you believe that diabetic complications and an early death are inevitable, you are likely to feel anxious, fearful, and depressed. You might bury your feelings and live for the moment, ignoring the measures that improve your odds. The idea creates the feeling; together they lead to inaction. When you believe nothing will help, you will do nothing to manage diabetes. Then—guess what?—you have a much greater chance of developing the complications you dread.

On the other hand, if you believe your actions will help, you can act to reduce the risk of complications and early death. You become more hopeful. Anxiety may still affect you, but you learn to handle it and maintain a positive attitude. When you do, it is much easier to follow a program and do the things that reduce your risks. Following your wellness program encourages positive feelings and helps prevent complications.

Beliefs and feelings affect actions, and in turn actions affect beliefs and feelings. Neither pattern is an inevitable response to having diabetes; either way, you choose the way you respond. You can become aware of your beliefs, feelings, and actions relating to diabetes and change them when they lead to negative results.

This is an incredibly powerful concept: you can change how you feel about an event or a situation. Once you identify its origin ("I am feeling upset because my blood sugar level was high and I thought I had taken the right amount of insulin"), you can tell yourself to put it behind you, that feeling upset is not going to help or change anything, and that you may as well feel neutral and go on to something else.

Change comes from seeking a deeper identity and detaching from seeing ourselves as our limitations. Not, "I am weak, sick, and unable," but, rather, "I am the person who can see these negative patterns without judgments. I am the person who chooses the life I live. I am the person who learns, grows, and changes. With this image of myself, I find it easier to use the information I have learned."

With a positive self-image as a foundation, you can work for specific change at the level of belief, feeling, or behavior. Or you may move from one level to another, integrating changes in beliefs, emotions, and actions.

Uncovering Your Beliefs

A belief is a statement about yourself or the world that shapes your life. It may be conscious or unconscious. Some beliefs give you power; some make you feel weak.

- I am capable of learning to manage diabetes; or
  I just can't manage—it's all too complex.

- Diabetes is a teacher, challenging me to be my best; or
  Having diabetes is a punishment.
- People accept me as I am; or
  People judge me for having diabetes and think I'm a bother.

Some beliefs restrict your ability to act and produce feelings of helplessness. Others are enabling, empowering, and encourage positive feelings. Limiting beliefs are often so deeply ingrained that you believe them to be true. They are reinforced by the feelings and actions that result from them.

If you believe you cannot control the amount you eat, your actions will prove you correct. You will feel depressed and eat even more to bury your feelings. The cycle can be broken by recognizing that beliefs such as these are not truths, but rather learned habits of thinking. When you view them as habits rather than facts, you reduce the power they have over you.

Many of your beliefs will be related to facts such as "people with diabetes have a higher risk of kidney failure than the general population." However, it is a mistake to believe "I will have kidney failure." A more appropriate belief is "I can act to reduce my risk of kidney failure." This belief is empowering and has a factual basis, because most people with diabetes do not develop kidney disease.

Watch for hidden beliefs as you learn about diabetes, especially at times when you feel stuck. Catalog the beliefs that empower you and those that limit you in your life with diabetes.

Techniques for Uncovering Beliefs

1. Ask yourself a repeating question: "What do I believe about (diabetes, home blood testing, complications, my diabetes self-care program, how diabetes affects my relationships, my doctor, my age)?"

2. Another way of doing this is to alternate between "What do I believe about?" and "What should I believe about?" Repeat the question for each topic a dozen or so times, writing down whatever beliefs come to mind.

   Example: What do I believe about myself as a person with diabetes?

   - I am more vulnerable than other people.
   - I should get special consideration.
   - I will probably die in my sixties.
   - My problems are a bother to others.
   - I am unwilling to follow a strict program; this is a sign of weakness.
   - Others should take care of me.
   - I really want to be fully responsible for myself.
   - I have learned to live better because of diabetes.
   - I value my life because I know how vulnerable I am.

3. In a concrete situation—especially at times of distress, frustration, or failure—ask, "What beliefs have created this problem?"

   Example: I have forgotten to take my morning dose of insulin or pills and don't notice the signs of high blood sugar until late afternoon. (I am scheduled for a job interview that day.)

   - If I'm sick, I won't be held responsible for anything.
   - Diabetes isn't really serious. I'm invulnerable.
   - Hurting my body is better than facing difficult challenges.
   - I'm weak and deserve to be hurt.
   - I want someone to take care of me.
   - I don't really want that job.

4. Choose an enabling belief you would like to adopt. Repeat it, holding out one hand as though it were speak-

ing the belief. Let the other hand state the limiting beliefs that oppose it. Keep repeating until you understand the conflicting beliefs and begin to resolve the conflict.

Right hand: A blood sugar test is free of judgments.
Left hand: It shows I've eaten like a pig.

Right: A blood sugar test is free of judgments.
Left: Big Brother is watching me.

Right: A blood sugar test is free of judgments.
Left: It makes me worry to see how high the test will be.

Right: A blood sugar test is free of judgments.
Left: Can I ever learn to control myself?

Right: A blood sugar test is free of judgments.
Left: I'd like to stop worrying so much.

Right: A blood sugar test is free of judgments.
Left: I really want to know the truth.

5. Write or speak a fantasy in which you are easily doing something that now seems difficult or impossible. Write down all the reasons the fantasy could not come true. Then write down the beliefs that would enable you to make the fantasy real.

After completing any of these exercises, underline the beliefs that seem most powerful, indicating those that limit you and those that free you. Then choose the limiting beliefs you would like to change.

Identifying limiting beliefs is the first step toward changing them. Awareness is often enough to dissolve the power a belief has over your feelings or behavior. However, you may have to take further steps to replace a belief with one that enables you to live as you wish.

Changing Beliefs

1. Create a positive phrase that clearly states the belief you want to adopt. Use your own words. Find ways to remind yourself that this new belief is entering your life (for example, put signs around the houses and repeat the phrase every day).

   Example: Replace the phrase "I can't follow my diabetes wellness program" with "I am improving my program step by step. I will continue until I have excellent control." The new belief is encouraging but not overwhelming.

2. Imagine yourself doing the things that would indicate you are living according to the new belief. Create a scene in your mind where you see yourself acting as you wish.

   Example: With "I am improving my program . . . " I see myself testing blood, keeping records, exercising, and doing other things that mean improvement for me.

3. Recall a scene from your life in which a limiting belief was active. Recreate the scene in detail, noting how the belief was expressed in your feelings and actions. Imagine how you would have lived the scene if you held the new belief at that time.

   Example: My old belief is "I must keep my diabetes a secret. I'll be rejected if people know." I'm embarrassed at lunch because a friend keeps insisting I eat her cake and I don't want to tell her I have diabetes. I'm afraid she won't go out with me if she knows. I get angry and uptight, and she is hurt.

   I want to adopt the new belief "I am open about having diabetes. Anyone who rejects me isn't worth having around anyway." I see myself at lunch, smiling

when my friend presses me to eat the cake. I say, "I've got a little secret I'm going to let you in on. I'd love to eat the cake but I really can't unless I take more insulin. I have diabetes." I sigh as she responds with surprise and caring. I answer her questions and feel relieved to have torn down that wall between us.

4. Trace the roots of beliefs and cut them. You learn beliefs from your parents or other people who have had a great influence on you. When you have trouble weakening a particular belief, determine who you learned it from. Visualize yourself giving it back to the source, or cutting the connection. With a belief specific to diabetes, you might have to look for an underlying belief.

   Example: I have a set of related beliefs: "I am more vulnerable than other people. I should get special consideration. I will probably die in my sixties." These beliefs are from my father, who had rheumatic fever as a child. He was sure he had cancer years before it finally developed. He was 67 when he died.

   I would rather believe: "I am both vulnerable and strong. I will give myself special consideration by living well. I will die when I die, and I can't predict when that will be." I see myself telling my father why I won't follow his example anymore. I give him a box containing his beliefs and he throws it into the fire. He smiles at me and says, "Go ahead. You are free to outlive me."

Handling Feelings

Many beliefs come from feelings. For example, the belief "I have diabetes. I'm going to lose my leg," may come from feeling afraid of being disabled. It can be tricky to change beliefs if you don't explore and deal with the feelings underneath them.

Also, living with a complex, life-threatening condition such as diabetes adds a lot of stress to our lives. The threat of long-term complications creates an underlying anxiety. A delayed meal, cut foot, or having no sweets available when blood sugar drops too low can be extremely upsetting. Identifying how we are feeling can help the stress to subside.

The following exercises will sharpen your emotional awareness and ability to work more effectively with your feelings. In this work, you may find strong emotions coming to the surface (particularly if you are dealing with a tough situation). If you do not usually feel things very deeply, this can be an alarming experience. You may want to talk about your feelings with a friend, support group, or professional.

What Am I Feeling?

1. **Breathe.** A very simple way of finding out what you are feeling is to sit quietly and breathe more deeply than usual. Feel your stomach, chest, throat, and face. Relax and breathe and allow the feelings to emerge.

2. **Imagine.** Visualize what you are feeling. Create scenes in your mind that act out your feelings.

3. **Move.** Let your body tell you what you're feeling by moving or dancing. Allow the movements to come spontaneously, without worrying about appearing graceful.

4. **Descend.** Often there are layers of feeling below the emotion you're conscious of. The experience of being caught in an emotion may stem from underlying feelings. Breathing, relaxing, and visualizing are ways to expose these deeper layers. After you've experienced each level, ask yourself, "What feeling is below this one?" Continue exposing layers to learn more about what you are feeling.

Just getting in touch with an emotion is often all you need to do about it. You may feel it for a time, express it, and go on with life. Other times, a feeling may seem eternal and inescapable. Perhaps you've just seen a relative with diabetes who has recently become blind, and you feel depressed. Or you've been on a food binge for two days and are filled with guilt and anger. If you're stuck in a feeling, try the tips below.

1. **Accept what you are feeling.** Don't compound the problem by chastising yourself for feeling the way you do. You have every right to feel whatever you are feeling. Use the techniques described above to explore this experience with a sense of curiosity.

2. **Express the feeling and communicate your emotions.** Draw, paint, write poems, speak to a friend (or into a recorder), sing, or dance. Communication often enables you to let go of a feeling that seems endless.

3. **Detach from the feeling.** Detachment is not suppression of emotion; it is a refocusing of awareness to achieve a broader sense of yourself. The emotion is present, along with your bodily sensations and perceptions of the world around you, as well as a self-awareness that observes the emotions, senses, and perceptions you experience.

Example: I am feeling hopeless and depressed. I can't escape this feeling. I feel the texture of the rug beneath my feet. My breath is shallow; my nose is dry as I breathe. I want to escape and go to sleep. I've never felt such deep despair. I see wind blowing trees outside the window; I hear the wind in the leaves. My stomach is tight. I smell the rose across the room. I hear music from downstairs; it's a song I like. My chest relaxes when I think of the words. Depression seems like a ball inside of me, instead of me locked inside it. The ball is dissolving. My breath is deep now. I have tears in my eyes. I'm alive again.

Creating Solutions

In order to become unstuck and solve a problem that is particularly troubling you, you need to become more aware of your problem and its source. The following exercise may help you.

Write a brief statement summarizing what you know about the problem you are facing. This summary will help you see the problem and identify the solution. Use the following questions for help.

Summarizing the Problem

1. What are the facts of your situation? Which aspects appear to be outside your control? Which ones are within your control?
2. When you examine how you are feeling about the problem, what are your strongest emotions? Where in your body do you feel them?
3. Consider your thoughts. Are there beliefs or attitudes that make you feel unwilling or unable to deal with this situation, such as "I can't cope with crisis," "It's too late for me to change," "It's not fair," "I shouldn't have to," "I don't want to."
4. What is it that you find difficult to do (or to stop doing)? Break down your behaviors into small parts. Figure out which is the hardest.
5. What pictures come to mind when you consider the problem? Do they help you understand what is happening?
6. Is there something you are holding onto by having this problem—some positive benefit, such as increased attention from someone you care about?
7. Is there something you are avoiding? What undesirable result might come if you were free of the crisis?

8. Is something else happening in your life that needs attention or is distracting you from what you are trying to accomplish with diabetes?

Some people are most comfortable doing this sort of work on their own, perhaps by writing in a journal. Others appreciate talking through a crisis with a friend or relative who is a good listener. A diabetes support group is another good setting for exploring such issues. If no progress is made in any of these ways, a few sessions with a counselor might help you sort things out.

Sometimes, a clear understanding of what is happening is all we need to get past an obstacle. "Oh, I was hung up on that old belief 'I'll die by the time I am 50,' just like Mom. No wonder I was stuck. It's time to get on with learning to live!" When this happens, tension is released and we can move forward.

This may be a time when you need **action**, not just understanding. If so, design the solutions to your problem. View the situation without blame or judgment. In the work you have just done, identify your beliefs, feelings, and behaviors that cause you stress and think of ways to deal with them.

Taking Action

1. Tell yourself that you can handle the situation. Recognize that you do choose your responses to what is happening, and you can make new choices.

2. Pay attention to your feelings, but do not be trapped by them. (Use relaxation or detachment, page 26, when negative feelings seem to dominate.)

3. Identify the realistic goals you want to reach. What changes will let you know that you are out of the crisis?

4. Brainstorm a list of actions that will help you move forward. Write down any ideas that come to mind, then search the list for those you feel prepared to take. Choose the one that will enable you to take a first step.

5. Imagine yourself taking the actions to overcome your problem. Let full-color movie scenes unfold in your mind in which you discover new answers. Don't forget the music.

6. Take a first step, no matter how small. Action gives you confidence to take another action and gets rid of anxiety.

7. Give yourself breaks, relaxation, and exercise. In most crises, you find solution in your time off.

If you do everything possible and still feel that you are getting nowhere, look for help from your health care team and personal support network. You don't have to do this by yourself. Some problems need outside input.

Another way to solve a problem is to tell yourself a story about it. This can help you pull together the threads of your beliefs, your feelings, and your actions so you can see how all three are interwoven. You can write this narrative or say it aloud to a friend or into a tape recorder. Use the most direct language possible.

For example, see Mary's story on the next page. By telling this story to herself, Mary can identify how her beliefs ("I have no self-control"), her fears ("I'm terrified I'll go blind"), and her actions ("I've been on a binge for two days") are all contributing to her problem of not feeling well. Mary gains perspective, understanding, and the willingness to change.

Mary's example focuses on a specific situation. You can also gain insight by telling your story in a more expansive manner. Describing your life with diabetes through the years can give you extraordinary perspective and understanding.

Mary's Story

I'm frustrated, angry, and guilty. I've been on a binge for two days and can't stop; I have no self-control. I'm probably taking years off my life when I do this. I must hate myself. I began eating Tuesday morning, just after Dr. Blast told me my tests were lousy and that I had to take better care of myself or I'd be in trouble. I've been trying hard and it doesn't seem to do any good. Nothing I do works out right. Why can't she understand how hard I've been trying?

Now I'm poisoning myself with candy and pastries. My blood sugar must be 500! Every time I eat something I feel worse. I'm angry at how weak I am. I'm afraid of what this is doing to me, and that I'll never learn how to take care of myself.

There was a blind woman at the newsstand in the lobby of Dr. Blast's building last Tuesday. I never even noticed her before then. I forgot about her right away, but now I can see her face so clearly. I'm terrified I'll go blind like her. I don't believe there's anything I can do; I can't do anything right.

No wonder I'm in such a mess. I must be stronger than I think if I can keep myself feeling this bad and acting so stupid for so long. My eyes are still fine and there's a lot I can do to keep them that way. Dr. Blast was worried and doesn't know how to be gentle. I can be gentle; gentle and strong.

—Mary, 52

You might do this with a friend who has diabetes or another medical condition, sharing stories at length.

When you have solved some problems and reached a level of achievement in your diabetes management, exploring how you got there both rewards and reinforces the changes you have made. Don't be bashful about giving yourself credit for living well with diabetes.

CHAPTER 3

16 Steps to Success

The biggest hurdle for me was accepting that I had diabetes. I didn't think I would get it, even though it's in my family. I thought if I ate right and watched my weight I would be fine. So when diabetes came knocking at my door I felt really betrayed.

I felt really depressed for a long time. Then one day I woke up and thought, you know, it's not the end of the world. Plenty of people have worse things. If I just learn how, I know I can feel well again.

—Lynn, 52

These steps to success will help you work any diabetes management program successfully.

1. Believe that treatment for diabetes is effective. If you doubt this, try to understand why you doubt.

If you believe anything about diabetes, believe this: keeping your blood sugar levels under control gives you the best chance of living a long, healthy life.

If you don't believe diabetes care will improve your health, you will have difficulty committing to any program. Go back to page 19 and explore your beliefs about diabetes.

2. Recognize that diabetes is a serious condition worth your attention, even if you have few symptoms at present.

When you have a moderate degree of control, you might not have symptoms of diabetes. Even when blood sugar levels are high, you can get used to short-term symptoms such as thirst, frequent urination, and sluggishness.

Unless complications develop, you might not understand the seriousness of diabetes through your experience with it. Unlike people with arthritis, for instance, you have few painful reminders. You have to create your own way of remembering that diabetes is a serious condition.

Writing down your thoughts can help you place diabetes in your life. Answer the questions quickly, even if the ideas that first come to mind don't seem to fit.

- What about diabetes makes it a serious condition that could have a major impact on your life?
- Do you ever feel you have no future because of the diabetes?
- Do you avoid looking at problems that arise because of your diabetes?
- Do you sometimes take diabetes too seriously? If so, how?
- Do you have any doubts about the seriousness of diabetes? (If so, see Chapter 11).

3. Balance seriousness with lightheartedness, detachment, and humor.

Diabetes is a lifelong companion, so you might as well make it an agreeable one, threats and all.

You can use lightheartedness when dealing with your situation. Speak of diabetes as though you are referring to another person, someone you are fond of and find gently amusing. Or visualize yourself and your dilemmas from the future where you have long since resolved them. Note the clever ways you avoided seeing the obvious situations back then.

Detachment is not "not caring," but rather viewing yourself and the problems you face from a higher place. From this point of view, you are not attached to the feelings and beliefs that often trap you. You experience and acknowledge them, but you realize that you are more than your feelings and don't let them limit you or what you can do.

Humor is a powerful way of breaking attachments. When you can laugh at your behavior, you feel less controlled by it.

4. Believe that you are able to learn and follow any program you choose.

Many people learn to doubt what they can do and what they set out to do. Whether your doubts come from feeling that you are dumb, weak, or stuck, you can learn to have a better self-image. Diabetes can make us feel dumb, no matter how well we learn about or change other areas in our lives.

5. Recognize that you are the one who chooses how you will care for yourself. Think about your decisions.

Your doctor, nurse, dietitian, social worker, or diabetes educator cannot make the actual choices for you. Only you can make them. You are the only one who can manage the prescriptions, diabetes-care recommendations, and external pressures in your life.

Ernie's Story

Out of 48 years of living with diabetes, I spent 30 of them trying to get it under control. I thought I knew what I needed to do, but actually doing it seemed harder than climbing Mount Everest. For one thing, I didn't feel I could ask my doctor for help. That meant I'd have to tell him how out of control I was! I always tried to look like a good patient.

So, I'd study my 1954 Joslin's *Diabetes Manual.* I'd measure the food I ate, pee in the test tube, get more and more uptight. Nothing made any sense to me. I couldn't predict when I would or would not spill sugar. An incredible sense of frustration and failure came with that stinking orange color foaming up at me in the test tube!

Of course, I always felt that I'd done something wrong, no matter how hard I tried. No one knew then that stress affects blood sugar levels strongly, or that urine tests aren't very accurate, or that one shot a day of intermediate insulin couldn't possibly prevent large ups and downs in blood sugar levels.

In short, I didn't know that I was in a double bind, being expected to do something but not having the tools necessary to do it. It was like being asked to build a house with bent nails and a hammer without a handle and feeling incompetent because the task seemed impossible.

Today the diabetes tool kit is full of new tools for both physical and psychological self-care. But, diabetes is still not easy to control. If you choose to work toward the highest level of control, your ability to learn and change behavior will be challenged. And in some cases, even with the best effort, a moderate level of control is the best that can be achieved. (It's still better for your health than not trying.)

Whenever you achieve less than your goal, don't label yourself a failure. Give yourself credit for what you have achieved, and look to see what you still have to learn to change to reach the goal. (This may be something other than what you set out to learn.) With this point of view, you learn from experience, and you continue to believe in your ability to learn.

—Ernie, 55

It can be difficult to accept the responsibility to make choices, especially when the choices conflict with what your provider recommends. You may find yourself saying, "I don't have time to do all this monitoring," or "The work cafeteria doesn't have the right kind of food for my diet," or "It's too much hassle to check my blood when I am at work," or "I carry enough stuff around with me already."

If you make your choices consciously and accept them, you gain power. ("I prefer to sleep an extra few minutes rather than get up to blood glucose monitor," or "I don't want to bother fixing a bag lunch.") Also, make it clear to yourself what other choices you might have. Then you may find it easier to make healthier decisions.

When you realize your power to choose all aspects of your program, then you are more likely to follow it. Your life is under control; you make the important decisions. If you rebel against your own authority, learning to stop becomes one more item on your learning agenda.

Your medical team can do more than recommend a self-care program. They can help you understand the options available to you, and work with you to identify and overcome barriers you encounter. Don't be afraid to say, "That's going to be hard for me to do because . . . ." Being honest with yourself and your team results in greater wellness, not less.

6. Make decisions about diabetes care with your other needs in mind. Don't neglect other important aspects of your life or the overall quality of your life.

Health professionals may place top priority on your diabetes care and may not talk to you about other concerns. Most of the time you need to balance your diabetes care with a host of other issues. If you don't, you might run into serious difficulties. Be sure to discuss your other concerns and get suggestions for how to care for them and your diabetes.

	Specific Need	Actions Called For
Family		
Leisure		
Other Issues		
Education and Intellectual Growth		
Spiritual Concerns		

Use the table above to list your needs and priorities. List important needs in the areas on the left, then use the other categories to help you rank them according to the amount of attention they demand from you.

If this exercise suggests that you have enough concerns to keep an army busy, don't despair. See what can possibly be postponed or dealt with gradually. Dedicate at least a few minutes each day to improving your diabetes care, even if it's a couple of minutes planning your next steps. In a month or two, set a date to review your priorities.

Several needs can often be satisfied by a single activity. Dancing or sports, for instance, can help you improve glucose control while providing enjoyment and social interaction. Better relations with your spouse and mutual support concerning diabetes issues could both be served by going to a support group or communications workshop. When you find connections between your different needs, you won't have to spend as much time dealing with them individually.

Difficulty	Urgency	Rank

7. When choosing how you will care for yourself, find a balance between your preferences and needs.

You can't ignore your feelings, but you can't let them dictate your decisions about self-care. The best choices come out of an inner dialogue between your emotional and rational sides, with help from intuition. This dialogue may just happen, or you may need something to guide your decision making.

One way of starting this inner dialogue is to write it out, including both emotion and logic. Write in two different colors. Then use a third color to select the best course of action.

8. Monitor your stress levels as you work on diabetes care. Use stress management tools to prevent your diabetes program from becoming an additional source of stress.

Try the relaxation exercises on page 185–187 or the stress management techniques on page 184–185. Be aware of when you're feeling stressed and do what works for you to relieve it.

9. Reward yourself for both your efforts and achievements. Recognize that feeling better is itself a reward for improved self-care.

As you work on learning and changing behavior, rewards help reinforce the effort you make and the changes you achieve. The greatest rewards come from feeling better physically and feeling more powerful mentally. Additional bonuses help keep your motivation high.

People often reward themselves with sweets or extra food, but for people with diabetes, this can be a penalty rather than a prize. How about creating a positive reward system instead?

Take a few minutes to write down a variety of rewards you would appreciate, such as gifts, good times, experiences, or things it would be nice to have. At the start of a diabetes learning project, promise yourself one reward for effort after a certain period, and another reward when you have successfully completed the learning project.

10. Define the tasks required by the program you choose. Divide the tasks and the behavior changes into small, concrete steps. Set goals that are detailed and clear about what you will do. Create a realistic schedule for the learning or change.

It may seem that learning to manage diabetes is a full-time job. That's why this step is so important.

When you divide a large project into small steps and schedule progress over a realistic period, the project becomes more manageable. Make the first step an easy one. No matter how much urgency you may feel, you simply cannot learn everything you need to know in one day. Once you have mastered the basic survival skills such as detecting and treating low blood sugar, administering your shot or other medications, and dealing with infections and illness, you can proceed with learning and making changes at a slower pace.

By setting reasonable and specific goals, you give yourself a much better chance of experiencing success. Saying "I'll get my diabetes under control sometime" is too vague. Aiming to achieve an average blood sugar test of 160 mg/dl in one month's time will give you a better target, and you will clearly know whether you have attained it. Be sure to set smaller goals that lead up to the main one, so that you can measure your progress toward your ultimate goals.

11. Explore possible difficulties you may encounter in the process of change. Plan ways of dealing with them in advance.

You may be one of the blessed few who never have trouble changing anything. However, most of us experience some difficulty when making changes. You probably know what troubles you've had in the past and how you dealt with them. By making some notes about what you have learned at the beginning of your diabetes education process, you will be able to apply creative solutions when you need them.

In the past, I have had trouble learning or following a diabetes program because:

____

I have run into trouble in areas other than diabetes because:

____

I have moved (or could move) through the difficulty by:

____

12. Make a commitment to changing your behavior and learning the skills and information you need. Sign a contract. Take a vow. Make a bet.

For some people, commitment to change falls into place easily, without being formalized. But others like to state their intentions in a way that helps them strengthen their will to change, in some cases by making a contract with themselves. If this appeals to you, you can use the following form.

A Contract with Myself

I commit myself to changing this behavior or learning this part of diabetes care (be as detailed as possible):

____

I believe this will improve my diabetes self-care by:

____

I believe I am capable of doing this, although I may need assistance in the form of:

____

If I experience difficulties in completing this task, I will:

____

I will receive the following reward for my effort on

______________________(date):

____

I will receive the following reward for achievement upon completion of ____________________ (fill in goal):

____

If I do not fulfill this contract, I will ____________________ (name a penalty)

____

I can reasonably expect to complete this by

____

____

SIGNATURE DATE

13. When you don't want to make a particular change, try it for a short time and see how it affects your life.

You may not want to make some changes in your lifestyle right now. When this happens, it helps to remember that we often exaggerate the consequences of changes we don't want to make. In our minds, we see only the negative side, and blow it up to monumental proportions.

If you do this, how about doing a trial run? For instance, go ahead and check your blood sugar four times a day for a few days, if that's what you're resisting. Make no commitment beyond this period. Then contrast what you actually experience with your expectation. Whatever the specific change is, you are likely to find that it's not as bad as you thought it would be.

If you still have trouble beginning, break the task down into smaller steps and try just the first step for a while, then try the second, and so on.

14. Give yourself positive feedback as you learn, and support yourself when you have difficulty learning. Let go of feelings of guilt or failure.

Having diabetes is an emotional strain. Don't make it a bigger burden by telling yourself you are handling diabetes badly. Improve your willingness to manage diabetes by accepting yourself when you have trouble learning about or following a diabetes program.

Don't ignore mistakes; observe them without blame. This is how we learn.

15. When obstacles arise, deal with them and learn from your experience.

Treat obstacles that you can't seem to overcome as new learning assignments. For example, if you have started to check your blood at home but are afraid to prick your finger, then your assignment is to learn to deal with fear, physical discomfort, and negative expectations. (New meters check blood from less painful sites, too.)

Perhaps the obstacle is resistance to learning about diabetic complications. Maybe you break into a cold sweat every time you think of the subject. In this case, recognize the opportunity to learn about your feelings of vulnerability or mortality. Before—and probably while—learning about complications, you need to work with these emotions. Perhaps you could enlist a friend, relative or other people with diabetes to help you.

16. Evaluate your efforts and achievements without criticizing yourself.

Each time you complete part of your diabetes learning program, take a moment to evaluate your work in a nonjudgmental manner. Look at how you worked on it and what you accomplished. Give yourself credit for what you have achieved, even when you have not yet reached your final goal. Be honest about the shortcomings of your work, but don't view the shortcomings as a sign of weakness. They represent valuable opportunities to learn.

The process of evaluation is important in learning to manage diabetes well. Our condition demands a great deal from us. There are many variables that affect diabetes control. Sometimes we can make the best possible effort and still blood sugar levels are outside the target levels. It is important not to add negative judgment to the frustration we naturally feel. To continue learning, we must congratulate ourselves for our accomplishments and look for the next step to take toward improving our diabetes management.

PART TWO

The Living Well Programs

CHAPTER

4

Choosing a Program

Having diabetes means having to make decisions about many things you never had to think about before. Making decisions that result in normal blood glucose levels requires information and skill, whether you have type 1 or type 2 diabetes. You need to be able to measure your blood sugar level at any moment; you need to be aware of the effects of food, activity, medication, and stress on your diabetes; and you need to know how to vary them to regain a healthy balance. Finally, you need support to maintain the thoughtful lifestyle that makes real control of diabetes possible.

Sometimes I get so confused about how to take care of myself. It seems like my doctor wants one thing, my dietitian wants another, and my wife wants something else. Whose diabetes is this, anyway? Don't I get to decide how I want to live?

—**Jack, 48**

Until the last few years, most of us were unable to achieve a good level of control. Once-a-day injections of intermediate or long-acting insulin could not provide the insulin activity needed to handle blood sugar rises after each meal. Diabetes medications for type 2 worked for some people, but not all. We knew little about the way emotional stress raises and lowers blood sugar. And the need for emotional support was scarcely recognized.

All of this has now changed. Home blood glucose monitors give readings of blood sugar levels any time we need them. An insulin pump or two to four insulin injections closely matches our body's natural needs. There are great new diabetes meds on the market. Changes in insulin dose, food intake, and physical activity can keep your blood glucose levels close to normal. We know more about how to deal with stress. And good emotional support networks exist.

So the time is right to learn to manage your diabetes effectively! But which living well program is right for you? Do you want the best control, also called tight control, which is available with the intensive program? Or is moderate control the best that you can do now, while you work toward tighter control? And what do we mean by control, anyway?

Most of us believe that living well is living with freedom. Yet when we have diabetes, we are told that we must control our metabolism, our blood sugar, and our eating. Sometimes it seems as though every aspect of our lives requires some kind of control.

One problem is with the concept of control itself. It doesn't sound like a very nice place to visit, much less live. No wonder controlling our diabetes often feels like a burden. Yet control is one of the most frequently used words in diabetes, and we have not been able to come up with many substitutes.

We can take away the word's negative meaning by thinking of the metabolic order, the health, it truly represents. When we work to gain control of diabetes, we are taking over a task our bodies previously handled in order to feel as good as we used to. We are cooperating with and helping direct our life processes. We are not simply managing diabetes; we are balancing our lives.

Does it matter if you have type 1 or type 2 diabetes as you think about control? No. Do people with type 1 need more control? No. Can those with type 2 "slack off?"No. Type 2 diabetes is just as serious a condition as type 1. The same complications can develop; in fact, some may already be present when type 2 diabetes is diagnosed. It is time for everyone—you as well as your physician—to take type 2 diabetes seriously.

There are more similarities than differences between type 1 and type 2 diabetes. The general goals for blood glucose management, as recommended by the American Diabetes Association, are the same for both types (see page 82; these goals may be adjusted depending on your individual situation). Tighter blood glucose control has the same benefits for people with both types of diabetes (see page 56). No matter which type you have, you can choose how much you wish to do to manage your blood sugar.

To achieve your goals, if you have type 2, you may need to lose weight (and keep it off) and increase your amount of regular physical activity. The good news is that losing 10–20 pounds (5–10% of body weight) or walking 15–30 minutes every day may be enough to make a significant difference. In addition, you may need to take a combination of glucose-lowering pills, pills plus insulin, or insulin alone. Because your body is still making some insulin, your treatment plan will help your body make even more insulin, make the insulin you do have work more efficiently, or both.

So many new tools are now available—primarily medications—that it is possible for almost anyone with type 2 diabetes to bring his or her blood sugar levels into the near-normal range. And achieving that goal will help you—and those with type 1—live well with diabetes.

Finding Your Current Level

How much balance, or control, do you currently have in your life with diabetes? We made up this questionnaire to help you find out. Circle the number that is most true for you. Your doctor's office can supply results of your lab tests. It's time to learn what your numbers are.

A. Level of Control

My last fasting blood glucose test in the lab or doctor's office was:	
less than 120 mg/dl	3
between 120–180	6
between 181–240	9
higher than 240	12
don't know or NA (not applicable)	7.5
My last A1C test was:	
less than 7%	3
between 7–8%	6
between 8.1–10%	9
higher than 10%	12
don't know or NA	7.5
My last test for LDL cholesterol was:	
less than 100	2
between 100–150%	4
between 151–200	6
higher than 201	8
don't know or NA	5
My average home blood glucose level when I check at least 1–2 times a day for the last 7 days is:	
less than 120 mg/dl	2
between 120–180	6
between 180–240	9
higher than 240	12
don't know or NA	7.5
If you do not check your blood, or if you do so less than twice a week, circle 12.	12
When you test for ketones in your urine, the test is:	
always negative	2
always negative unless I am ill or under stress (or I have type 2 and I rarely test)	4
occasionally positive (1–2 times a month)	6
frequently positive (1+ times a week)	8
don't know or NA	5

I have had severe low blood sugar in the last month (strong symptoms such as confusion, sweating, shakiness, or pounding heart):

never	2
1–4 times	4
5–10 times	6
more than 10 times	8

I have been unconscious from a reaction or failed to awaken to a reaction occurring during sleep in the last year. If yes, circle 16. If no, skip to next question. 16

I have had symptoms of high blood sugar (frequent urination, nighttime urination, thirst and no energy) in the last month:

never	2
1–3 times	4
4–10 times	6
More than 10 times	8

I am normal weight	3
I am slightly overweight (up to 10% above normal)	6
I am moderately overweight (10–20% above normal)	9
I am very overweight	12

I seldom have illness or infections, and I recover or heal easily when I do	1
I have occasional illness or infection, and I recover slowly when I do	3
I am frequently ill and have infections, and I heal slowly	4

My energy level is good and I recover from exertion easily	1
I occasionally feel lethargic	2
I tire very easily and need to rest frequently during the day	4

In the last year I have been hospitalized because my diabetes was out of control:

never	4
once	9
more than once	16

B. Level of Program

I am on an intensive program (3 or more injections per day, using both rapid-acting or long-acting insulin or the insulin pump) and vary dosage according to blood sugar checks	3
I take two injections per day, but rarely vary dosage from day to day	6
I take only one injection of insulin each day	9
NA	6

In the last two months I have forgotten or deliberately not taken insulin or diabetes meds:	
never	4
1–2 times	12
more than twice	16
NA	10.5

I check blood glucose levels 2 or more times a day	3
I check blood glucose levels at least twice a week	6
I check blood glucose levels at least once a week	9
I seldom (or never) do any home blood checks	12

When my blood sugar is high or low or when there are changes in my routine (schedule, activity level, food intake, or stress), I know how to change insulin, food, or activity to match the changes. I can return to normal quickly	2
I make some general adjustments, but do not get back to normal for a few days	4
I know when my control is off, but I rarely do anything about it	6
I don't know anything about adjusting insulin, food, or activity to maintain control	8

I measure or can honestly estimate the amount of food I eat. I eat a balance of carbohydrate, protein, and fat	3
I usually eat moderate servings and have a general awareness of the amount of carbohydrate, protein, and fat	6

I eat pretty much what I want, but not to excess	9
I frequently eat excessively or irregularly	12
I seldom eat sweets or other sweet carbohydrates (such as dried fruits and fruit juices)	3
I eat small portions of sweets and other sweet carbohydrates	6
I usually eat small portions, but I binge at least once a week	9
I eat all the fruits and sweets I want	12
I eat as little animal fat as possible (butter, fatty meat, luncheon meat, and high-fat cheese)	3
I almost always eat only small amounts of animal fat	6
I usually only eat small amounts of animal fat, but at least once a week I binge	9
I eat all the animal fat I want	12
I eat healthy carbohydrates and high-fiber foods (whole grains and vegetables):	
at most meals	2
about half the time	4
rarely	6
never	8
When I have eaten too much or know that a large meal is coming, I use extra insulin or exercise to balance the extra calories:	
nearly always	2
usually	4
rarely	6
never	8
I do moderate to strenuous physical activity regularly	2
I do moderate physical activity, but it usually varies quite a bit from day to day	4
I am seldom active	6
I am not active	8
When I am under emotional stress, I cope well, and the stress does not seriously affect my blood sugar level	2

I try to cope, but my control may be off for a few tests 4
I don't cope too well, and my blood sugar level may be high for a day or more 6
I forget everything I know about coping, ignore my diabetes, and my blood sugar stays high 8

Add up the numbers you circled for parts A and B and enter your totals here:

Part A: Level of Control __________

Part B: Level of Care __________

Now check out your level of control and level of care. Your score should give you a sense of where you are and what you need to work on.

Level of Control	Score
Optimal	34–42
Moderate	43–65
Loose	66–90
Barely there	91+

Level of Care	Score
Intensive	28–42
Moderate	43–63
Loose	64–84
Barely there	85+

These ranges are taken from the authors' experience.

Completing this exercise can be challenging, perhaps even unpleasant. If your results are not as positive as you thought they would be, don't blame yourself. Acknowledge the choices you have been making and the reasons you have been making them. Give yourself room to begin making new choices. You might go through the program part of the questions and check the places where you marked the higher numbers. These will indicate areas for improvement and management that you may feel willing to begin at this time. A little later in this chapter, there is another exercise that will help you choose the overall level of management you wish to exercise.

Defining the Choices

Given all the benefits of tight control (see page 56), you might think it should be the only choice offered to people with diabetes. It is the best choice, but diabetes care is just one of the things we must manage in our lives. Once you try out the moderate and the intensive programs you'll know how much flexibility you can gain by following one or the other.

Begin at a level you feel comfortable with and then proceed toward tight control. It is better to have at least some control of your diabetes than none at all. The choices you make about diabetes control show in your day-to-day actions. Every day, you are the person controlling your diabetes, not your doctor or health care team. Support yourself in the choices you make, and keep working toward best control. The new experiences and skills you master will bring you to this higher level sooner than you expect.

The Moderate Program

This program is a place to begin to learn how to take care of yourself. It doesn't protect you as much as the Intensive Program but it gets you on the right road. The moderate program consists of:

1. Regular home blood sugar checking (monitoring) at least once daily, and as needed to figure out the cause of highs or lows.
2. Diabetes pills and/or insulin shots daily, usually with a combination of rapid-acting and intermediate or long-acting insulins. (The insulin pump is not recommended with this

program because you need more frequent blood sugar checks.)
3. An A1C of 7 or less.
4. Knowledge of food choices and carbohydrate counting and ability to follow a meal plan for reasonable body weight and blood sugar control.
5. An active lifestyle, a regular exercise program, or both.
6. Ability to make small adjustments in medications, food intake, and activity level to balance blood glucose.
7. Knowledge of the role of physical and emotional stress in diabetes and the ability to manage both in healthy ways.
8. Commitment to continue diabetes learning and meet your emotional needs.

The moderate program differs from the intensive program in the level of feedback and control it provides. Blood glucose monitoring is less frequent and, as a result, your insulin and/or pill dosage is set and can't be adjusted. It is less flexible than the intensive plan.

Home blood sugar checking is an important part of this program, even if you only do it once a day. Seeing your results helps motivate you to improve control. Having a meter on hand means you can easily see how stress, a large meal, or an unusual level of exercise affects your blood sugar. When you are ill, you can handle blood sugar and ketone problems more accurately. If you have difficulty detecting low blood sugar, you can use the checks to confirm it and become more aware of its symptoms.

Sometimes, success in improving control dramatically increases your motivation. If you feel that you could never handle the intensive program, you may find that beginning to improve management gives you greater willingness to try it. You will feel much better about yourself than if you just continued believing that you could never control your diabetes.

The Intensive Program

This program can help you achieve nearly normal blood sugar levels in a few weeks to months. The intensive program consists of:

1. Blood sugar checking at least 4 times a day (as many as 6–8 times a day at the beginning). For those with type 2 diabetes, checking is 3–4 times a day (more frequently in the beginning), and at different times each day to determine blood sugar levels overnight and before and after meals.
2. An A1C of less than 7%.
3. For type 1, insulin shots 4 or more times a day, often both rapid-acting and intermediate or long-acting insulins, or by insulin pump. For type 2 diabetes, work with your health care team to determine the best combination of diabetes pills and/or insulin.
4. Knowledge of food choices and carb counting and ability to follow a meal plan for normal body weight and good blood sugar control.
5. An active lifestyle, regular exercise program, or both.
6. Ability to adjust medications, foods, and activity level for changes in blood glucose.
7. Knowledge of the role of physical and emotional stress in diabetes and the ability to manage both.
8. Commitment to continue diabetes learning and meet your emotional needs.

The staples of diabetes care are all here—insulin, pills, meal plans, physical activity—but we've added several new ingredients. In this approach, frequent glucose monitoring allows quick feedback about blood sugar levels, which enables you to make more precise decisions about medications, activity, and food. For people with type 1, multiple insulin injections or the pump provide a level of insulin matched to blood sugar levels and amounts of carbohydrate eaten. For people with type 2, adjusting medications, food, and activity allow you to achieve near normal blood sugar levels over a 24-hour period.

Awareness of the effect of stress on diabetic control helps you understand puzzling swings in blood sugar levels. Stress hormones raise blood sugar, but you may not be aware of when you are under stress. You need to become aware and learn ways to relieve or manage the stress, which help reduce these swings.

Benefits of the Intensive Program

There are so many benefits to the intensive program!

1. You're much less likely to develop complications. Research has proven that the better your control, the less likely you are to develop long-term complications of diabetes. Good blood sugar control can delay or prevent the development of diabetic retinopathy, nephropathy, and neuropathy in people with type 1 and type 2 diabetes. Even though participants on the intensive program in one famous study did not reach normal blood sugar levels, their risk of complications was reduced up to 70%, and every step toward normal helped!

2. You feel better emotionally. As soon as you begin the learning process to achieve tight control, you may feel better. Many people report a sense of greater power, less depression, and less anxiety. This emotional high helps you through the initial learning period. Once you've mastered the program, you'll experience even greater freedom. You can deal with changes in food, mealtimes, activity, and stress, and still have nearly normal blood sugar levels.

3. **You feel better physically.** When your blood sugar levels are closer to normal, you simply feel better. You have more energy; you need less sleep; you are less likely to feel tired. Your immune system works better, so you are less likely to become ill or have infections that get out of control. When you do become seriously ill, you are better able to deal with the effect of the physical stress on blood sugar, and you are less likely to develop ketoacidosis. You will have many fewer hospitalizations.

4. **Your sex life may improve.** With healthier blood vessels and nerves, men reduce the risk of impotence. Women in good diabetes control develop fewer vaginal and urinary tract infections and consequently may find greater enjoyment in sex. It is vitally important to have tight control before and during pregnancy to reduce the risks for both mother and child.

5. **Children grow and develop normally.** For children, good diabetes control encourages normal growth and development. Growth is sometimes stunted when blood sugar is poorly controlled in childhood. Fluctuations in insulin requirements caused by growth spurts and the hormonal changes during puberty are more easily handled in the intensive program. This program provides children the best route to a healthy adulthood.

6. **Other important body functions become normal,** such as elements in the blood that are responsible for clotting, levels of cholesterol and triglycerides that contribute to heart and circulatory disease, the release of certain hormones, and the thickness and fragility of capillaries (the thinnest blood vessels). These functions don't operate well if you have high

blood sugar. They are the building blocks from which diabetic complications are constructed over time.

7. **If you already have complications, good control will slow or stop their progression.** In some cases, complications may be reversed or their impact lessened by careful management. Whether or not existing complications can be reversed, your chances of avoiding or slowing the development of other complications is also improved. The immediate physical benefits and the emotional lift gained by taking control help you better deal with the fears that usually accompany the diagnosis of complications. See your doctor before starting a more intensive diabetes program if you have complications.

Costs of the Intensive Program

What are the costs of better control?

1. **Lifestyle changes.** You have to be more aware of your meal plan, activity level, and daily schedule. (Anyone who wants to be healthy must do this.) If you have not been taking very good care of yourself, the changes can feel substantial, but once you commit to trying them, you gain more freedom in your choices.

2. **Money.** The cost is higher, because you measure blood sugar more often. Your insurance may cover monitoring supplies. Meters can cost $50 to $200, but discounts and rebates often lower the cost almost to free. Your diabetes medication costs money, but you'll be saving money on doctor visits since you'll be healthier all over.

3. **Time.** During the first months of intensive management, there is a cost in time and energy. Collecting information about yourself, keeping records, and figuring out what the records mean can be a major project, but it is no more com-

plex than learning to drive. Once you know your patterns and what to do, your time is free for other things.

4. **Organization.** You need to organize the parts of your life that affect blood sugar, which will simplify the tasks and save time. The more you do this, the more quickly you will reach the point where you do not have to be so organized. It is much easier to learn how to keep your blood sugar within limits if you follow set routines during the training period. Without these routines, it is difficult to know what is causing your blood sugar to be too high or too low. Once you establish a routine, you'll enjoy much more freedom.

5. **Hypoglycemia.** If you have type 1 diabetes, you have a higher risk of low blood sugar episodes while you adjust this program. (This is less likely if you have type 2, but still possible.) This is especially true if you have usually had high blood sugar levels or follow an irregular exercise or meal plan. (Often, fear of lows is one of the reasons some people with diabetes keep their blood sugar high.) You need to sharpen your awareness of the cues indicating that a low is on its way, and **always** have some form of carbohydrate with you. You can easily check with your meter whether those funny feelings are the result of low blood sugar or some other cause, such as anxiety. (For more on handling low blood sugar, see Chapter 10.)

Weighing the Costs and Benefits

Take a moment to consider how the costs and benefits of better control balance out for you.

- What values do *you* place on these benefits?
- Which are the most important to you?
- Do any of the costs seem particularly heavy?
- If so, what could you do to lighten them?

Who Needs the Intensive Program?

Everyone needs this program! Some people choose this path because they want to live as healthfully as possible and avoid complications. Others will make this choice because of a specific and immediate health need such as a healthy pregnancy and baby. The intensive program is especially recommended for:

- Anyone who wants to be as healthy as possible.
- Women who are pregnant or planning to become pregnant.
- People who don't want to develop diabetic complications such as nerve and kidney disorders, circulatory problems, heart disease, retinopathy, and other eye disorders. Tight control can slow these down, too. (If retinopathy or kidney disease has started, see your doctor.)
- Children whose growth is significantly behind schedule.
- People with other chronic illnesses or conditions, where the consequences of high blood sugar make the other chronic conditions worse.

Who Doesn't Need It?

There may be medical reasons for not following this path. You and your doctor should weigh the pros and cons. Because of the increased likelihood of low blood sugar, patients with heart disease or stroke on this program might be adding too much risk. Patients with advanced kidney disease have less predictable insulin action and may find the intensive program difficult to manage.

You may need your own blood glucose targets if you have difficulty recognizing the symptoms of low blood sugar. This is also called hypoglycemia unawareness. After living with diabetes for many years, the usual signs of low blood sugar can diminish or disappear because of hormonal changes. Your doctor can study your blood glucose records with you to determine whether this has happened to you. You may need to sharpen your awareness of the physical signs of low blood sugar. Medicines for some other condition (such as beta blockers for high blood pressure) can also lower your ability to recognize symptoms.

If personal obstacles are making it hard for you to try this program, you may wish to seek assistance such as individual counseling or a support group. If you decide to continue with a moderate program for now because of other problems, review your decision later to see if a different choice is possible.

Selecting the Right Program for You

If you have not decided which level of program to follow, answering these questions may help you do so.

1. I need to achieve improved control soon because:

- ☐ I want to reduce my risk of complications.
- ☐ I have diabetic complications.
- ☐ I am pregnant.
- ☐ I am planning to become pregnant.
- ☐ I am a child whose growth is significantly below normal.
- ☐ I have another major illness.

2. I should be cautious when moving to an intensive program because:

- ☐ I do not experience the usual symptoms of low blood sugar and it is difficult for me to detect it.
- ☐ I have significant kidney disease, heart disease, risk for stroke, or blood vessel disease.
- ☐ I have beginning diabetic retinopathy or nephropathy.

3. The reasons I have for wanting to improve my control of diabetes include

____

____

____

4. Other major problems that need my attention are

____

____

____

5. I could gain assistance and support in dealing with these issues by

____

____

____

6. Could I postpone working on any of these to gain time for diabetes?

____

____

____

7. The external supports I now have for dealing with diabetes are:

☐ great
☐ enough
☐ not enough

8. In making decisions, I also have to consider

____

____

____

Review your answers, discuss them with your doctor and those close to you, and then choose a living well program you can be happy with.

9. Given the above, my choice of program is:

☐ moderate
☐ intensive

CHAPTER 5

The Moderate Program

While tight control is the goal for everyone with diabetes, there are some reasons for choosing a moderate level of control. For some, starting with the moderate program still represents an enormous improvement in diabetes management. (While it is not the best care, it is better than no care!) For others, it is a fall-back position. Look at this program as one step along a continuum of diabetes care and blood sugar control, ranging from no care to best care. You can move from one to the other and back again, depending on what else is happening in your life. Diabetes care is always evolving; and the decision you come to today about diabetes care can change tomorrow. With the moderate program, you can find a place on the continuum and begin to learn what to do to be healthier as you move toward tighter control.

I want to take care of myself, but I want to do other things too. It's hard to change habits at my age. I just want to do the basics right now, enough to feel good and prevent future trouble.

—Cindy, 58

We know that every little bit of improvement in blood sugar control helps. Good control provides you the best chance of avoiding complications. It is important to have the best control possible, but not everyone is ready for the intensive program. Some people are more comfortable with a moderate level of control until their motivation is boosted by an event like the onset of a complication. Most see the moderate program for what it is, a temporary treatment plan until they are ready for a more detailed approach.

Whatever your reasons for selecting the moderate program, it is important to allow yourself the most basic ingredient of living well—accepting your decision for now. The intensive program is praised so highly that you may feel a bit anxious, perhaps even guilty, about choosing "second-best." Feelings like these are not good for your health. Yes, it is important to keep working toward best control, but encourage yourself along, don't waste energy worrying.

Your decision to follow the moderate program was not made in isolation. You weighed your needs both as a person and as a person with diabetes, your motivation, and the support available to you. The moderate program seems to you to be the wisest choice. Live well with it today, but revisit your decision often to see if tighter control is possible for you.

As you work with this program, you may find your interest in self-care growing, or you may streamline your diabetes case in a whole new way. Simply having the immediate feedback of blood glucose testing may improve your control and increase your motivation to manage your diabetes. You may move toward improved control just by learning the information and skills needed at a pace that is right for you.

You may feel anxious because you are not ready or willing to gain optimal control right away but you want to avoid developing complications. Many of us have experienced anxiety about developing complications. It was something we lived with, consciously or unconsciously, but now we know that there are positive things you can do to handle it (see pages 167–169). The moderate program may reduce your risks of complications, but it won't do as much for you as the intensive program will.

10 Steps to Program Success

If you've chosen the moderate program, follow the steps below.

Step 1: Be sure you have a positive setting for your diabetes learning, a diabetes management team that agrees with your goals, and support from family, friends, and other people with diabetes.

It's time to review and strengthen your learning foundation. A key helper is, of course, your physician. You need one who is well informed about the newer approaches to diabetes care and who knows that you play the leading role in diabetes management. Your doctor should work with a diabetes educator and dietitian and other team members as needed. Discuss honestly what you are doing with your doctor and set guidelines for the decisions you make at each step. Most doctors, nurses, and dietitians are pleased to see their patients taking greater responsibility for their own diabetes, and support your independence fully. Some of them discuss test results and special problems by phone and provide 24-hour access in case of emergencies. Ask about this if your doctor doesn't suggest it.

The encouragement of your family will help you during this time. Let the people close to you know what you are working on and what it means to you; share your concerns and expectations. Ask for the help you need to change any family patterns that interfere with your efforts to improve management. If you are in a negative family situation, you will need to take some action to neutralize your family's influence and look for support from others.

You should let your friends know about your goals and ask them for assistance. This is very helpful when you are attempting to make basic lifestyle changes. Friendships often revolve around habitual behavior and may be threatened when you begin changing habits. Instead of meeting friends to eat, you might prefer to walk and talk. You can reduce the "threat" to others and gain valuable aid if you communicate the importance of the changes you are making. They'll get healthier too, if they join you. Realize that some friends may be too attached to their old image of you; if they offer little support, let that be their problem, not yours. Keep moving.

Finally, remember the support and guidance you give yourself when you feel stuck, frustrated, confused, or discouraged. It is likely that you will reach this point one or two times in the coming months; it is a natural part of the process. While you are still full of enthusiasm, plant the seeds for the times when you may forget how creative you are. Review your strengths and skills. You might write a note to yourself to open when you feel that you can't go on. Remind yourself of your accomplishments when you feel you haven't made enough progress.

Step 2: Get lab tests of A1C, kidney function, blood pressure, and blood lipids (triglycerides and cholesterol) that show your present level of control.

The A1C, kidney function, and blood lipids (fats) tests will allow you to see how effective your self-care has been to this point. The A1C test measures your blood sugar level over 2–3 months. Kidney tests tell you if high blood sugar levels have damaged the tiny blood vessels that filter blood. Blood pressure tests tell you more about your risk for heart disease.

The lipid tests tell you if you are at greater risk to develop complications and/or heart disease. High levels of cholesterol or triglycerides often appear along with high blood sugar values. Their presence over long periods contributes to the development of diabetic complications. These blood fats are also major contributors to the development of heart and blood vessel disease, conditions which affect people with diabetes at a rate two to four times greater than people without diabetes. Your blood lipids should be tested at least every year to see if they are in the normal range.

You and your doctor can set goals for these tests that are reasonable. Then, new lab tests, along with your own feelings of well being, will be the best cue to how you are doing. You will find that the feedback from the tests will be very helpful, although at first you may need guidance from your doctor or diabetes educator in interpreting them.

Step 3: Learn the skills and information needed for the moderate program, including how to check blood sugar and urine ketones and how to recognize and treat low blood sugar.

Self blood glucose monitoring is the greatest advance in diabetes care since the discovery of insulin. It provides accurate information about the level of your blood sugar. With this information, you can make decisions regarding insulin dosage, exercise, food intake, stress, and reactions. It is one of the keys to achieving both the best diabetes control and greater freedom in your life.

The technology has improved greatly in the last few years, providing finer, gentler lancets and user-friendly meters. New meters check blood from forearms and thighs, which is painless. The new meters are faster, smaller, and much more automatic. The more often you check your blood, the better information you'll have to manage your diabetes.

To ensure the accuracy of your readings, it should be at least 60°F, or breathe on the strip while the blood is on it to keep it warm. Many of the newer strips are usable over a wide temperature range—check the information that comes with them. Use the sides of your fingertips; they are less sensitive. Use a large enough drop of blood so you don't have to smear it on the strip (the blood should stay liquid). Some of the newer strips, allow you to add more blood if the initial drop was not enough. Don't use gauze to remove the blood (it may scrape off the test material). Some new meters don't even use strips. Never use the test strips after they have expired.

If you are still reluctant to monitor your blood sugar, see if you agree with any of the objections listed below.

- **"I'm afraid it will hurt."** You may already be sticking yourself at least once a day to take insulin, yet your fingertips seem more sensitive than your thighs and upper arms. Use the sides of your fingertips. When it is adjusted to the proper depth, you almost never notice when the lancet strikes. The anticipation of the pain is usually worse than anything you actually experience. It is a good idea to rotate from finger to finger, to keep any one spot from getting too sore. You might try a newer meter that samples blood from forearms or thighs, which is not painful.

- **"Won't it be terribly expensive if I start testing several times a day?"** You can lower costs in two ways. First, buy strips from a discount mail-order firm. Second, if you have health insurance, check if monitoring equipment and supplies are covered. Most medical plans are now picking up these costs.

- **"Won't I get discouraged if I see too many high results?"** You probably will, but deal with the discouragement by remembering that this information is important in learning to control your blood sugar. High tests indicate that you have more to learn, not that you are weak or unable to control yourself. Use the checks to increase your motivation to master the program.

- **"How often do I have to check?"** Curiosity may lead you to check frequently at first. It is satisfying to be able to determine the exact impact of food, activity, or stress on your blood sugar levels. Check as often as you can but at least 1-2 times a day.

- **"I can tell whether I'm high or low by how I feel."** This is true only if you have very high or very low blood sugar. Usually, you cannot sense much without actual symptoms. You may be able to learn to sense blood sugar levels in the midrange by using the feedback from your blood checks. For a few weeks, write down your guess before checking. Then see what the meter says. You'll find the meter can give you much more reliable feedback.

- **"Can children handle home blood monitoring?"** Children can certainly do it, with the proper support and guidance of adults. (It helps if the adults stick their own fingers or forearms and check their own blood a few times to offer encouragement and a good example.) Four- and five-year-olds have learned how, though they are usually a few years older before they start doing their own monitoring. In fact, once they are trained in monitoring, children become excellent instructors of their peers and older adults.

If you're on insulin, the best schedule for the moderate program is to check your blood sugar before taking your morning insulin, before meals, and at bedtime. The daily fasting blood sugar check allows you to supplement your morning shot with rapid-acting insulin to balance high readings when they occur. Starting the day in control helps you stay controlled throughout the day. The other checks tell you how well you maintain control throughout the day. If you aren't on insulin, try to check in the morning and before meals.

If this is more checking than you are willing to do, determine a schedule of checking that you feel able to follow consistently. Checking once or twice a day is better than nothing. Keep a log and schedule checks at different times each day so you can see the pattern of results throughout the day—before and after meals—when you look at your log for several days.

By starting to check regularly, you will create a good habit for the rest of your life. Even once daily checking can help you improve control to some extent. Some people find it helpful to make a contract with themselves or their doctor or diabetes nurse, stating the number of checks they will do. Then they share their results with the doctor or nurse at the next visit.

You should do additional blood glucose checks when illness upsets your control and to check your symptoms of insulin reactions. Sometimes you may mistake symptoms of anxiety and stress for those of low blood sugar. To become more comfortable with blood glucose checking take a class if one is available, or have your doctor or diabetes educator instruct you in the correct procedures. Get yearly tune-ups to your technique.

Your doctor can give you your own target blood glucose levels. Or ask your doctor if the target blood sugar levels in the box might make sense for you.

When your blood sugar is high (greater than 240 mg/dl) testing urine for ketones provides important feedback. Ketones in your urine indicate that your diabetes is getting out of control due to insufficient insulin (too much food, not enough insulin, or too much physical or emotional stress). It is especially important to check for ketones if you are ill (even with a bad cold), especially if you are nauseated or vomiting and cannot keep food down.

Your average blood sugar level over the past 2–3 months can also be indicated by an A1C test. The A1C test measures

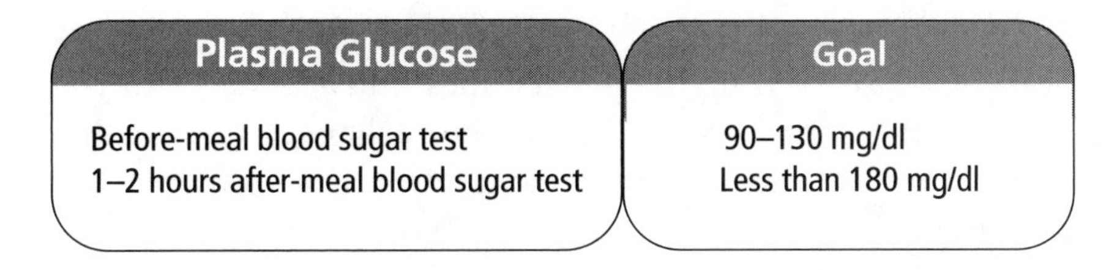

Plasma Glucose	Goal
Before-meal blood sugar test	90–130 mg/dl
1–2 hours after-meal blood sugar test	Less than 180 mg/dl

the amount of sugar bound to hemoglobin in your blood over time. For example, if your A1C is around 9%, your average daily blood sugar was probably about 240 mg/dl. If it's 10%, your average was about 275 mg/dl, and if it's 12%, your average was 345 mg/dl. The A1C goal in this program is under 7%.

Anyone working to improve his or her control of diabetes should also control blood pressure and cholesterol levels, too. The target levels are in the table below.

Step 4: Determine how regular your meal plan, activity level, and daily schedule will be.

Without several blood checks a day to guide you, you are more likely to have low or high blood sugar levels if you do not follow a fairly regular meal plan, activity level, and daily schedule. (The intensive program, on the other hand, allows much more flexibility, once you are past the first two or three months needed to learn it.)

Ideally in the moderate program, you stick to a fairly consistent and healthy meal plan, using either the exchange system or carbohydrate counting, and eat on a fairly consistent

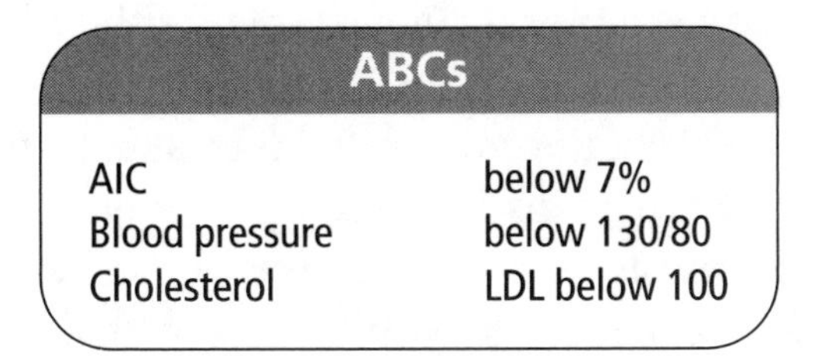

ABCs	
AIC	below 7%
Blood pressure	below 130/80
Cholesterol	LDL below 100

schedule (not more than an hour off schedule unless you know your blood sugar is high). When a meal must be delayed, you should eat a snack and deduct those exchanges or carbohydrates from the meal when you eat it. Physical activities should be fairly regular from day to day, as you adjust your insulin dosage or food when there is an increase or decrease in the amount of exercise. As you gain experience with these adjustments, you may find it possible to increase the flexibility of this program.

It is up to you to decide how much of a schedule you can tolerate. Fortunately, the combination of your home blood checks and the A1C test in the lab will tell you if your decision allows you to maintain a moderate level of control over a two- or three-month period. If your A1C test is too high, you will know that you need greater regularity. Work with your doctor or diabetes educator to find the places where you can tighten your program.

Step 5: With your doctor's guidance, establish your ongoing medication and/or insulin plan.

There are now five different classes (groups) of medications to treat type 2 diabetes. Each class acts differently in your body and has its own pros and cons. Your doctor will help you find the right pill or combination of pills for you. For more information on the different diabetes pills available, see Appendix 3, pages 236–237.

Many people with type 2 diabetes delay going on insulin because they are afraid of the needle. In the meantime, their AIC climbs and high blood sugar damages their body. If your AIC goes higher than 8, despite your best efforts, try insulin and see how much better you feel. To be successful, you need to know the pattern of insulin activity—when it begins, when it peaks, and how long it is effective, which you can see in graphs on the next page. Ask your doctor which insulins might be best for you.

Insulin Type	Onset	Peak (hours)	Duration (hours)
Rapid-acting			
Aspart	Less than 15 minutes	1–2	3–6
Lispro	Less than 15 minutes	1–2	3–6
Short-acting			
Regular	0.5–1 hour	2–3	3–6
Intermediate-acting			
NPH	2–4 hours	4–10	10–16
Long-acting			
Glargine	2–4 hours	Almost flat	Usually over 24
Ultralente	2–4 hours	10–16	18–24

Figure 1. Insulin levels before you had diabetes

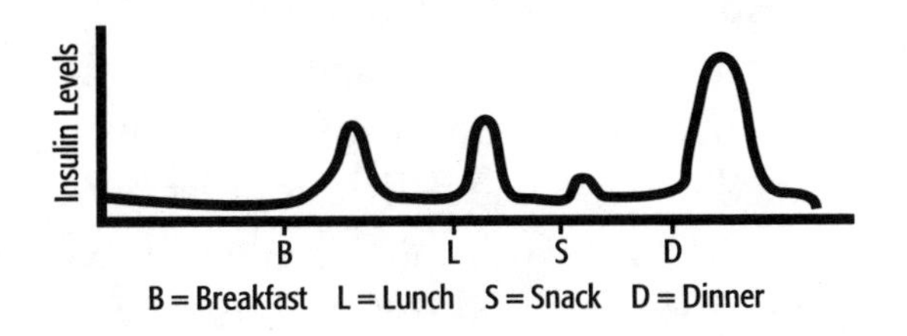

Figure 2. Insulin Plan: Glargine Plus Rapid-Acting

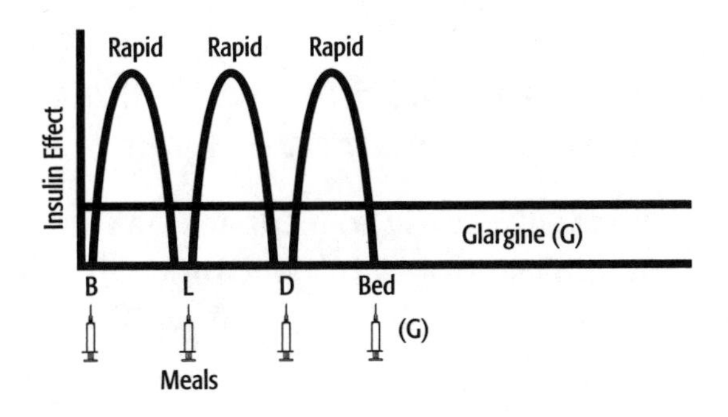

People with type 2 still have some natural insulin in their bodies and may only need one shot of long-acting insulin a day. Work closely with your doctor or diabetes educator at this stage, identifying patterns by studying your records. Your doctor will try to develop a plan so that insulin activity matches your lifestyle and physical needs.

Step 6: Observe the changes in your blood sugar level caused by stress, illness, changes in food and exercise, and other factors.

Keep a record of your blood sugar checks. You won't believe how much you can learn about your unique response to changes in your routine. There are many different influences on blood sugar levels. If you keep careful track on a log like the one on pages 92–93, you can use that information to understand your daily and weekly diabetes records. Seeing your blood sugar levels swing up and down and not knowing why they change can be frustrating. But if you keep thorough records for a few weeks, you can quickly learn to recognize some of the reasons for your fluctuations.

You'll learn to vary insulin dosage, food, and exercise cautiously to compensate for high or low levels and to deal with changes in your daily routine. With understanding, you gain more power to control your blood sugar levels. Read the story on the next page to find out how one woman handled her daily fluctuations.

Step 7: Have lab tests done after two or three months to determine the effect of your new program.

At this point, you will have solid feedback on the effectiveness of your regimen. Tests for A1C and blood lipids, together with your home records, will let you know if you have found the right balance in your program of self-care. As you review the results with your physician, be objective. You have certain target levels you want to achieve. If you haven't reached them, don't judge yourself, and simply look for the reasons. The next step will help you do this.

Sandra's Day

Sandra, a working mother with two children, notes in her record the glargine she takes before breakfast. She usually snacks in the afternoon and before bed. When she ate too little carbohydrate at breakfast, Sandra found herself with low blood sugar before lunch, so she ate two doughnuts to be sure she wouldn't go low again. Too many doughnuts, a usual amount of lunch, a missed exercise session, and the stress of a business meeting increased her blood sugar too high.

She knew that her blood sugar was fairly high, so she checked and noted that it was 240. She skipped her afternoon snack and she ate a very light dinner. When she checked 2 hours after dinner, her blood sugar was high in spite of reduced carbohydrates and an evening walk with the kids.

When she checked her blood sugar at bedtime, it was still high, so she skipped her bedtime snack. The next morning, her blood sugar was within her target range. By cutting back on food and taking a walk, she had been able to cut the high blood sugar down to size.

Step 8: Assess your progress. Find out how to further improve your control or maintain the level you have achieved. If you have not achieved all of your goals, identify obstacles and how to overcome them.

Give yourself some credit! No matter what you have achieved so far, the fact that you are still at work means a lot. If you feel like it, create a "hanging-in-there" award and give yourself a special treat.

Go through the previous seven steps that you have been working on. See which ones you have completed and which ones need more work. Make sure you haven't missed any. Again, give yourself credit for what you have done and don't blame yourself for what needs to be done.

If you find that you have learned all you need to achieve a moderate level of control, take a moment to review the decision you made on the living well programs. When you consider all factors, is a moderate program still your choice? Knowing how much better you could feel with tighter control, is it time to move on to the intensive program?

If so, you have already accomplished a major portion of what you need to learn, so it will be much easier to make the transition. Check the chart on page 82 to see how the intensive program is different. The main changes will probably be checking your blood more frequently, possibly changing medication or insulin plans, and fine-tuning to adjust for the variations you observe. Discuss the necessary changes with your doctor before proceeding.

Step 9: Stay motivated and continue to work on improving control.

If you choose for now to continue at the moderate level, or if you still have more to learn about this level, keeping your motivation high is important. It may have been an easy process so far, or it may have been frustrating. Either way, you will need to take steps to encourage yourself and remain willing to continue.

Support from other people with diabetes who are also working on improving control is one of the most important ways to keep motivation strong. If you have not yet found ways of obtaining support, it is time to do so. Support groups or individual contacts can give valuable emotional support and encouragement. You can receive practical guidance from people who have overcome the obstacles you may still be struggling with. You may also help others with problems you have already solved. Helping others is good for you, too, and keeps your motivation high. (See Chapter 13 for more on getting and giving support.)

Any program is easier if you do not feel you are serving on "active duty" every day of the year. Occasional breaks or vacations can be part of your program. Don't feel that you are cheating at these times. A day or two of relaxed management can make it easier for you to continue with your usual level of control. If you take supplements of rapid-acting insulin to handle any feasts, be sure to match the insulin to the carb to avoid severe lows. (Such vacations are not advisable if you have any infection or a complication that could be made worse by higher blood sugar levels.)

If you have significantly improved your control, you are probably feeling better, both physically and mentally. This quick payoff makes it easier to continue following your program. It also becomes an inspiration for continued learning. This is reinforced by the blood checks, too. When you can see exactly what your blood glucose level is—and do something about it—you gain power over diabetes, instead of feeling controlled by it. It is natural to want to extend this sense of power by learning more about how to manage your condition well.

If you ever feel a strong resistance to continuing with your program, there are steps you can take to explore and neutralize the issues that are getting in the way. Be aware of any rationalizations or denials that you use to justify the resistance. Don't accept "I'm really too busy" or "I don't need to be so careful, I'm all right now," or "It won't do any good anyway." Use the processes on pages 20–22 to gain awareness of what is happening and ask for help if you need it.

Step 10: Celebrate!

When you understand the moderate program, you have completed a challenging assignment. You may feel like honoring yourself for your achievement, privately or even publicly, with a party, dinner, or picnic. Whether you invite a small group or a large one, give yourself credit for the many things you have learned. What you are doing to live well with diabetes makes you well all over. Other than taking insulin and checking blood, the basics of your regimen are healthy for anyone. So share the health.

Now is the time to collect a reward if you promised yourself one to build motivation at the beginning. In fact, even if you haven't made an agreement with yourself, go ahead and treat yourself to some special thing, event, or experience. Living well is its own reward, but there is nothing wrong with a special treat from time to time.

You may have chosen to stay at a moderate level of control while you dealt with other aspects of having diabetes. You may find that you have learned enough to continue gradually improving your blood sugar management while also focusing on other issues. Possibly, there are new problems or challenges in your life that you need to handle while you take a break from diabetes learning (perhaps applying in other areas what you have learned about yourself here). If so, make a date with yourself to reopen the subject in two months or so. Mark the calendar "time to start learning more about diabetes" or "time to start working on tighter control." Diabetes is a lifelong companion; you will benefit from seeing it as a lifelong teacher.

On the other hand, now that you have mastered the moderate program, you may be eager to go right on to the intensive program. You now have a solid foundation of knowledge, so this will be easier than it would have been a few months ago!

Is the Moderate or Intensive Program Right for You?

The moderate and intensive programs are very similar in construction. They are different mainly in the degree of control over blood sugar levels, as the chart on the next page shows.

The intensive program aims for tighter control over blood sugar and lower A1C tests. This calls for more frequent monitoring of blood sugar so you can use more frequent insulin shots or an insulin pump to mimic the way the body naturally controls blood sugar levels. Both programs have similar meal plans and exercise schedules.

Task	Moderate	Intensive
Blood sugar monitoring	Once a day, or as often as you are willing to test	4 or more times/day
Blood sugar goals		
Before meal	90–130 mg/dl	90–130 mg/dl
Max after meal	180 mg/dl	180 mg/dl
A1C goals	Less than 7%	Less than 7%
Insulin use	Set doses of pills or insulin or combination	Insulin doses change based on: 1. carbs 2. activity 3. blood glucose level 4. patterns
Meal plan	Consistent carbs at the same times of day	Carb counting Insulin: carb ratio

CHAPTER 6

The Intensive Program

> You know, from what I've seen so far, this isn't so hard. It's like going to school. There's a certain body of information to learn, and then steps to take, like solving math problems. I like doing calculations and figuring out how to keep my blood sugar level on track. And I feel so good—like I'm in charge.
>
> —Joe, 24

You learn much more easily when you divide large projects into smaller steps. You can see each task more clearly, and see progress toward your goals. This is especially important when you start to learn the intensive program and make the necessary lifestyle changes. How you learn the program can make the experience safer and more useful. You may already have some of the required skill or knowledge, but we urge you to review all of the information in this book. You may learn something you haven't seen elsewhere.

11 Steps to Optimal Control

Step 1: Create a positive foundation. Be sure you have a good doctor, diabetes health care team, or diabetes educator who agrees with your goals, and support from family, friends, and others with diabetes.

You are starting one of the most positive and challenging things you can do for yourself as a person with diabetes. The rewards for you on physical and emotional levels are great, indeed! You will have to overcome obstacles to gain these rewards. Your first step is to make sure that the foundation for this work is positive. This includes creating realistic expectations, neutralizing past failures, organizing professional and personal support, and becoming familiar with the things that you can do to keep going.

First, realize that learning this program will take some time. You just can't flip a switch and gain instant control. The process takes one to two months, and sometimes longer. Guard against becoming discouraged. Some people often follow the intensive program perfectly and improve their control, but still experience large fluctuations in blood sugar levels.

If at first you don't succeed, find out what else you can do. Discuss what is happening with your doctor or diabetes educator; be patient with yourself and give yourself credit for what you have achieved. Sometimes improving diabetic control requires a stress management class, couples counseling, or a less stressful job. A different insulin may be needed to overcome immunity that can develop after years of injections. If you have type 2 diabetes, a new medication or combination of medications or adding insulin can help you gain better control.

Support from others with diabetes, especially those that are also learning the intensive program, is second only to the guidance of your physician and diabetes educator during this period. Individual contacts or a support group can offer you encouragement and reinforcement, and practical tips on the details of management. Some physicians organize a buddy system or support group for people working on improving control. Such groups can also be organized by individuals working on their own, with a diabetes educator, or through your local American Diabetes Association chapter.

If it is necessary to step down your degree of control, spare yourself the additional stress of feeling guilty. Respect your decision and keep the postponed changes on your agenda to return to as soon as you can.

Learn ways to protect yourself against "permanent" failure. One way is to see setbacks as temporary. You are not failing; you just have something to learn before you can succeed. Although you may feel a sense of urgency about learning, it is helpful not to be too judgmental and hard on yourself. Transform obstacles into a part of the learning process by letting them define the next lessons you need to master.

You may have to set aside a history of frustration and lack of success. In the past, perhaps you did not have the tools you needed to achieve your goal. Let go of the feeling "I'll never get this right." You can do it—if not now, then soon!

The fear and sense of urgency that inspire many to learn the intensive program need to be balanced with more positive motivation. Fear is a powerful feeling that can move us for a time, but our progress is steadier and more lasting when it comes from a positive sense of being good to yourself.

Step 2: Have lab tests taken to provide a benchmark of control.

Lab tests can give you an accurate picture of your present level of control. These usually include A1C, fasting glucose, and blood lipids (fats, triglycerides, and cholesterol). The A1C test tells you how your blood sugar level has been over the past 2–3 months. The blood lipid tests tell if you are at greater risk of developing complications and/or heart disease.

The results of these tests, along with your other records, tell you where you are and where to go to obtain better control. More importantly, they can tell you how far you have come. The feedback you receive when you compare the next set of lab tests with these results may be very encouraging. Or, if there is little improvement, the new tests will help you determine what to do next.

Step 3: Learn the early skills and information necessary for the intensive program.

- **Learn how to do accurate blood sugar checks.** With this feedback, you can tell when you need extra insulin (or less food) and how much. You know when you are going too low, and you do not mistake the symptoms of an anxiety attack for those of low blood sugar. You know the effect on blood sugar level of a particular meal or snack, or a period of exercise. By making conscious decisions about this information, you can guide your body to a level of metabolic control that is near normal.

  Precise feedback about blood sugar levels has an impact on your behavior. It becomes easier to deal with the craving for a hot fudge sundae when you've seen your blood sugar shoot up to 450 mg/dl after eating one. A much-postponed stress management class becomes a high priority when you've seen a distressing day at work produce a record high in blood sugar. With home blood glucose checks, you have a tool for understanding how you live with diabetes. You begin to understand the reasons for the highs and the lows, and you begin learning how to do something about them. That's living well!

Your doctor can give you individualized target blood glucose levels. You may need to work for months to achieve these levels. Don't despair—every little improvement is well worth the effort. With time and practice, you'll come closer to your goals.

For the first month or two of the intensive program, you may need to check 6–8 times a day to understand your patterns of response. This includes checks before each meal, at bedtime, and, sometimes, two hours after a meal. That feedback will tell you how the food you have eaten has affected your sugar level. You can refine your skill in using your intuition, symptoms, feelings, and blood monitoring to predict how different foods will affect you. Knowing this, you will be in a better position to choose what to do to achieve your target blood sugar levels.

- **Learn how to recognize and treat low blood sugar (hypoglycemia).** This skill is so important that we have devoted an entire chapter to it (Chapter 10), which you should read regardless of what you may already know about hypoglycemia. The symptoms will change when you follow the intensive program. When your metabolism is well controlled, your symptoms become more subtle and difficult to recognize. Or you may have more frequent reactions. Make sure you know how to increase your awareness of early symptoms of lows (see page 157) and how to prevent severe nighttime hypoglycemia.

- **Test your urine for ketones.** In the intensive program, urine testing is useful to check for ketones when your blood sugar is high. Keep ketone test supplies on hand, for when you are ill or stressed. Ask your doctor what you should do if you find ketones in your urine. It will include drinking no-carb liquids and taking small doses of rapid-acting insulin.

- **Keep careful records.** Keeping precise records that you and your doctor can learn from is as important as checking. Record your blood sugar tests, food, activity level, and stress. (Once you establish good control, you may be able to keep less detailed records.) During this period, you are a scientist studying your own metabolism. The information you gather will help you learn about your own patterns of response. (For more on recordkeeping, see Step 5.)

Step 4: Make routines for meals, exercise, and daily schedules during the learning period.

Organizing your life will give you much more freedom in diabetes management over the long term. While learning the intensive program, you should follow a careful meal plan and maintain a similar exercise level each day. Eat the same number of calories, carbs, or food exchanges in each meal and snack; and maintain a similar activity and exercise level from day to day. Also, maintain the same medication and/or insulin dosage until your doctor advises you to make changes, and don't vary the timing of shots or meals by more than one hour.

Without this step, it will be difficult to understand how your system responds to the different factors affecting your blood sugar level. If your food intake, exercise level, daily schedule, and stress exposure change each day, you lack the solid information you need to establish the best medication plan. Without dependable results, it will be difficult to vary insulin or other meds, food, and exercise to balance blood sugar levels that are too high or too low.

After a month or two of following this routine, you can be more flexible and still maintain good blood sugar levels. You will have learned how your system functions, how the different aspects of your program affect you, and how to vary them to obtain good control. You will also have learned some internal signs that alert you to your level of control. You will understand what has caused a high or a low, and you will have the ability to make changes to balance the highs and lows. Thus, a relatively short period of following a schedule will give you greater long-term freedom.

This does not mean you should become compulsive about your schedule and create new stress in your life. Keep things as regular as possible from day to day, and observe how changes in food and activity affect your program. (Remember, the best learning is guilt-free.) Allow yourself to take a day or two off from the routine now and then; you will return to it with renewed energy and dedication. The changes you make will last if you achieve them because you want to rather than you have to.

Some people find it difficult to follow a schedule, whether because of outside demands or their own emotional reactions. Work schedules and levels of activity change frequently; daily exercise may not fit into busy lives; or you may want to retain your version of freedom.

Even if you find it difficult to make your life more systematic for a few months, you can still improve your control. Check as often as possible and record the results. Review these records with your doctor or diabetes educator to get a better idea of what makes your blood sugar rise and fall. By doing this, you will be more willing to try for greater control because the effects of your lack of routine will be apparent.

One way to make this period of increased regularity more acceptable is to offer yourself a reward. For some, the benefits of improved control are reward enough. However, others need to reinforce their motivation by giving themselves a special gift or experience. After so many weeks of following a strict program, you become eligible for that trip or event or object you have been wanting. And you can plan for smaller rewards as you reach new milestones along the way. Keep moving!

Step 5: Begin a period of frequent checking and recordkeeping. Keep detailed records, and observe how you respond to your present program.

Many of us experience a sense of excitement as we begin checking blood sugar at home. For the first time, we are able to observe how our system is affected by food, exercise, inactivity, and stress. We can determine if a queasy feeling is low blood sugar, stress response, or merely an unexpected queasy feeling. We can measure the effect of a few cookies or extra slices of bread and butter. We have the feedback essential to living well and maintaining diabetic control.

In the beginning your doctor or diabetes educator will probably ask you to observe your blood sugar readings without making any changes in your program. You will need to keep records for several days, along with detailed notes on food, exercise, stress, and any changes that might affect your blood sugar.

During this initial period, you will learn the most if you check before every insulin injection, before each meal, one to two hours after each meal, and at bedtime. Also, check your blood sugar when you suspect that you are going too low. If you think you have nighttime low blood sugar, set your alarm and check at 2:00 or 3:00 in the morning.

This may sound like a lot of checks (up to seven or eight a day), but checking this often is necessary for only a few weeks, and the information you gain is invaluable. With it, you and your diabetes team will be able to tailor your medication and/or insulin, food, and activity to achieve a high level of control.

It is useful to assume the role of scientific observer, rather than as judge of right and wrong, as you record your results. You are likely to find the swings in blood sugar level puzzling at first. It is easy to believe that you have done something wrong. However, you will learn faster if you simply record the results (even if it is the result of a binge) and move forward, without blame. Record all of your checks; don't skip any because you know they will be high. This will help you understand how high they actually are. You are in the process of learning to control blood sugar; you can't possibly have everything under control already.

Try the sample daily log on pages 92–93. Other logs provided by meter and insulin companies are also available. Record your results under "Blood Sugar." When you miss a check, indicate your estimate (for example, "low," "high," or "150.") Include lows in the blood sugar column, with the amount of food used to treat it in the food column. Grade lows as mild (1), strong (2), or severe (3). Indicate the type of insulin if you use more than one.

Under "Meds/Insulin," record what you take. Grade "Activity" for each period of the day relative to what is normal for you at that time: 1 = no activity, 2 = less activity than usual, 3 = your normal level, 4 = more activity than usual, 5 = maximum activity. Include how long you did each activity.

Under "Food," indicate carbohydrates or exchanges and anything out of the ordinary, such as delayed meals. If you calculate only carbohydrates, indicate over- or underconsumption. Also, note the particular foods you ate and the results of your post-meal check.

Under "Comments," include potentially stressful events, whether or not you felt an emotional response. Note difficulty with sleeping, periods of tension or relaxation, worry or anger or emotional highs, and physical occurrences such as illness, menstruation, or low energy—anything that can help you explain the variations in your tests.

Daily Diabetes Log

Date/Time	Blood Sugar	Meds/Insulin

Activity	Food	Comments

Remember, these records are useful not only to your doctor or diabetes educator; they are most valuable to you. Analyze and learn from them, and make changes based on what you learn. By recording this information, you can see the pattern of your life with diabetes.

Step 6: With your doctor, select your medication and/or insulin plan.

By using the information from your blood sugar checks, you and your doctor can decide what medication and/or insulin plan would be best for you. Make the adjustments needed to obtain the highest possible level of control. If you have type 2, consult your doctor to see if your meds should be changed or insulin added or adjusted. For more on common diabetes medications, see Appendix 3, pages 236–237.

How Insulin Works

The effect of insulin on your blood sugar level depends on many factors. Below are some of them. Variations in any of these factors can cause changes in your blood sugar level.

1. The type(s) of insulin you use, and the level and schedule of your dosage. The type(s) of insulin you use determines the pattern of insulin activity in your body throughout the day. A rapid-acting insulin can begin acting as soon as 5–15 minutes following injection and reaches its peak 1–2 hours afterward. Long-acting background insulin, on the other hand, has very little peak with a duration of 12–24 hours (page 75).

Each type of insulin has its characteristic profile of action (page 75). Often, rapid-acting insulin is combined with intermediate or long-acting insulin to create a series of insulin peaks. These are matched to mealtimes and a "basal" level to accommodate the body's ongoing needs for energy as shown in these graphs.

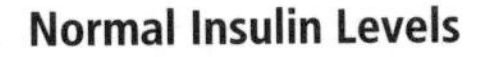

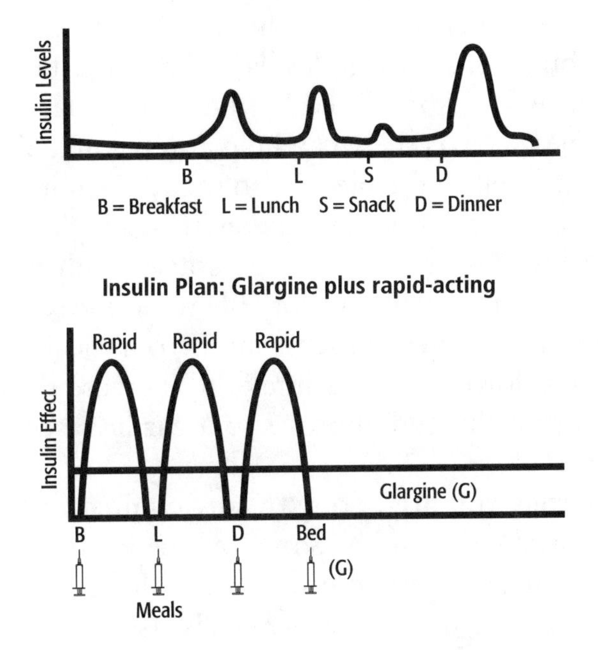

2. The site of the shot. Where you give your insulin shot may affect the timing of its action. For example, insulin injected into an arm that will be swinging a tennis racquet or legs that will be running will quickly activate the insulin injected into them.

3. The timing of the shot in relation to your meals. Rapid-acting insulin, such as lispro, can be taken 0–15 minutes before you eat. If your blood sugar is high, you might take it an hour before you eat and check to be sure your glucose has come down before eating. If you are low, you might eat first and then take your insulin.

4. Your current blood sugar level. The ability of insulin to lower blood sugar is decreased by high blood sugar levels. At normal levels (70–110 mg/dl), one unit of rapid-acting insulin will usually lower blood glucose 30–50 mg/dl. With a higher level (over 120 mg/dl), it might take three units of insulin to lower it by the same amount. This is one reason blood sugar levels can skyrocket and remain high for several days. If stress or a food binge pushes high levels and the usual insulin dose is taken, its effect is inhibited by the excess sugar. Extra insulin at times such as these can help you regain balance.

High fat levels in the blood also reduce insulin's ability to lower blood sugar. You might experience a high after a meal unusually high in fat but not necessarily high in carbohydrates, because the insulin is not able to do the same amount of work in the presence of excess fat. If your meals are high in saturated fat, lower your fat intake to increase the effectiveness of your insulin and improve your cardiovascular health.

5. **Other drugs you are taking.** Many common prescription drugs interact with insulin. Some reduce insulin's ability to lower blood sugar or otherwise increase blood glucose. These include diuretics, drugs for heart disease and high blood pressure, and estrogens or steroids that increase glucose production in the liver. "Beta blockers" may be particularly troublesome because they minimize the usual signs of low blood sugar—sweating and rapid heartbeat. The over-the-counter drugs most likely to influence blood sugar are decongestants and antihistamines. Ask whether any drugs prescribed for you can affect your insulin use or blood sugar level, especially when you go to a doctor other than the one you see for your diabetes. Use your blood checks to determine whether you should change your insulin dosage while taking the prescribed medication.

6. **Adjustments.** By the time you have established your insulin plan, you will understand the timing of each insulin component—when it peaks and what meal it covers. The timing of reactions will help you understand your schedule. You will also be able to make adjustments in dosage to keep your blood sugar within the target range you have established.

If your activity level changes significantly from weekday to weekend, you will need to adjust dosage to account for the change. Women will need to make adjustments when menstruation affects blood sugar levels. Workers with swing or graveyard shifts will also have to adjust their insulin. In the beginning, check with your doctor before making such changes. As you become experienced, you will be encouraged to take the initiative.

Sample Insulin Plans

Different insulin plans involve multiple injections each day, mixtures of different types of insulin, or the continuous infusion of insulin provided by the pump. Your AIC and daily glucose checks will tell you which works best for you.

1. Two shots of intermediate and rapid-acting insulin: one before breakfast and one before dinner. The peaks of the rapid-acting insulin handle the increase in blood sugar caused by breakfast and dinner. The peaks of intermediate insulin handle your lunch and overnight needs. Greater convenience is the major advantage of this plan. The disadvantage is that you have less flexibility in the timing and size of lunch. If your checks are high at midday, you might need an extra shot of rapid-acting insulin to cover lunch.

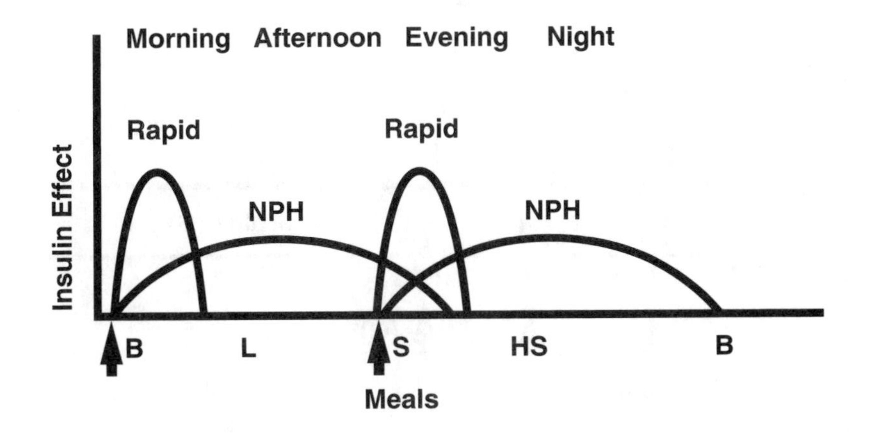

2. Three shots: intermediate and rapid in the morning, rapid before dinner, and intermediate at bedtime. This allows better overnight coverage if you need more low-level insulin action while you sleep, so you can wake up to normal blood sugar levels. But this plan doesn't allow much midday flexibility.

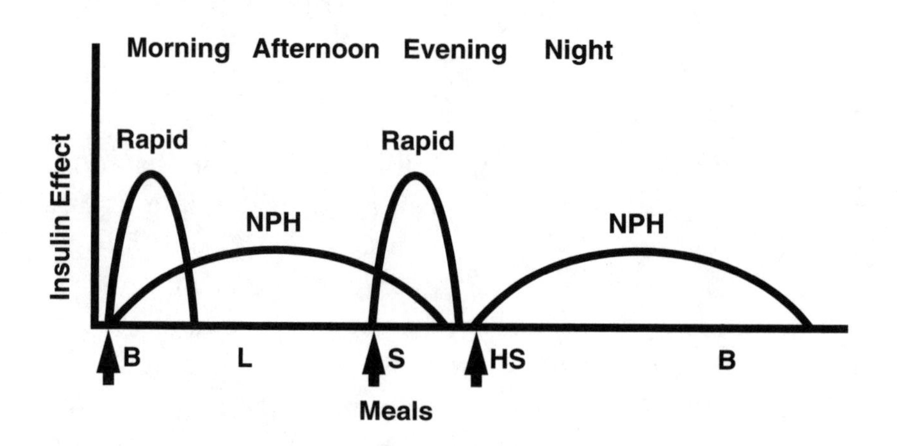

3. Four shots: rapid before meals and long-acting at bedtime. This plan allows you to adjust dose according to meal size. The long-acting insulin before bed provides low-level insulin action throughout the night and next day.

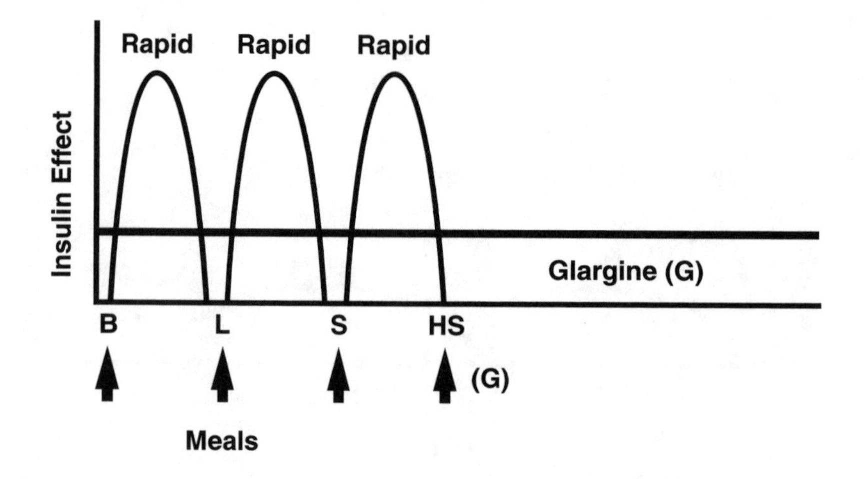

4. The insulin pump provides both a continuous low-level flow of insulin (basal) and bursts (bolus) before meals. The insulin pump comes closest to the natural pattern of insulin availability found in people without diabetes. The device pumps a small amount of insulin at regular intervals under the skin (usually in the abdominal area) through a tube and needle (called a catheter) that remain implanted day and night. This is the "basal" insulin rate that can be adjusted to match the metabolic rate of an individual. Before a meal or snack, you trigger a measured burst or "bolus" of extra insulin to handle the increase in blood sugar from the food. These measured bursts are also used to lower blood sugar when it is too high.

You usually change the site every two to three days. The needle is removed immediately after insertion, leaving behind a soft, flexible tube. This allows short-term disconnects without the need for inserting another needle set. You need to check your blood sugar 4–7 times a day to adjust premeal boluses to balance blood sugar levels. You also need to watch for low blood sugar and the danger of sudden increases in blood sugar due to crimping of the tube or a rare pump malfunction. With only rapid-acting insulin in your body, dangerous highs can happen quickly when the supply is cut off.

Some people dislike shots and resist the idea of taking several a day. Insulin pens, prefilled disposable ones or those loaded with insulin cartridges, can make multiple injections more convenient and user-friendly. They are easy to carry, easy to use, and inconspicuous. Most people who try them continue to use them, especially for shots away from home. An alternative to shots with a syringe is jet injection. This is a needle-free method that administers insulin at a high pressure through the skin's surface.

When you take two or more shots each day, you can adjust the peaks of insulin activity and insulin availability to meet your needs. In fact, this individualization is essential. Your doctor will use your blood sugar records to determine blood sugar levels throughout the day and explain what to do when the levels are high, so you can take action to bring blood sugar down.

Things to Know about Insulin Use

You may experience some of the following problems as you work with your insulin plan.

- If you have a major improvement in control at this stage, and the majority of your tests are in the target range, you might feel physically uncomfortable for a short time. You may even have symptoms of hypoglycemia when your blood sugar levels are normal. This is natural while you adjust to the new level of control. The discomfort can last up to two weeks. When your system adjusts to the new level, you will feel better that you ever did when your blood sugar was chronically high.
- If it is difficult to bring your tests within the target range, or if there is a great fluctuation in your readings, don't despair. There can be many reasons for the fluctuations you experience, and there are just as many solutions. Work on figuring out causes and solutions instead of blaming yourself.
- A frustrating aspect of insulin therapy is getting high blood sugar levels soon after treating your low blood sugar. Take care not to eat too much carbohydrate. In addition, one of the body's responses to low blood sugar is to release the hormone glucagon, which releases glucose from the liver. That glucose, plus the carbohydrate you use to treat the reaction, means you can have high blood sugar levels within an hour of hypoglycemia. Hypoglycemia caught in an early stage usually doesn't produce this increase.

Occasionally, you will have low blood sugar during the hours while you're asleep, when you can't detect low blood sugar. The body's natural response may bring blood sugar to a level above normal by the morning check, and you may increase your insulin. High levels before breakfast can also be caused by the normal physiologic predawn rise in blood sugar called the "dawn phenomenon."

If you have near-normal 3:00 a.m. blood sugar levels (which you can set an alarm to wake you so you can check) and high pre-breakfast blood sugar, you probably have the dawn phenomenon. If you have near-normal bedtime blood sugar, low-normal or hypoglycemic 3:00 a.m. blood sugar, and high pre-breakfast blood sugar, you may need a bedtime snack or an insulin adjustment. If all three levels are high, you probably need more insulin. Ask your doctor more about how to treat these situations.

Step 7: Observe variations in your blood sugar level caused by changes in food, exercise, stress, illness, and other factors.

You will start to observe the causes of blood sugar variations as soon as you begin checking. By now it will be easier to determine what is causing a particular high or low reading. Read Chapters 8, 9, and 12 to learn more about how food, physical activity, and stress affect your blood sugar. Your doctor may want you to spend more time observing before you begin making changes to compensate for levels outside your target range. Or you may begin making changes right away.

The skills you learn in this step are central to improving blood sugar levels while maintaining a flexible lifestyle. When you are able to vary the ingredients of your program, you are able to live with a degree of freedom not previously experienced by people with diabetes. You can bring blood sugar levels back to normal within a few hours when they are high, and easily handle the effects of illness or emotional stress. You can change schedules, food intake, and exercise and still maintain your target levels. The decisions you make are part of a balancing act that used to take place automatically before you had diabetes.

There are two types of changes you will be making on a daily basis: those that compensate for levels that are too high or too low, and those necessary to prepare for a change in routine. The feedback from your checks will teach you exactly how much you should adjust insulin, food, or exercise to produce a change in blood sugar level. At first, change only one element at a time so you can determine what effect the change has. Later, you will be able to change more than one aspect at a time.

Work with your health care team to determine how to make the right changes for you. In general, if your blood sugar is too high, you can increase rapid-acting insulin, increase exercise, or decrease carbohydrate intake. If your blood sugar is too low, you can increase carbohydrate intake or decrease insulin. To prepare for extra activity or exercise, you can decrease insulin (rapid acting or intermediate) or increase carbohydrate intake.

Step 8: Have new lab tests done to measure the effect of your new program and to establish ongoing goals.

After you have been on the intensive program for two to three months, your physician will order new A1C and blood lipid tests and will probably want to review your daily logs. The logs provide objective information concerning your level of control. With it, you and your doctor can determine if any further changes in program are needed.

At this point, you will establish how often to do blood glucose checks and what level of recordkeeping to maintain. One study found that control suffered if people checked fewer than three or four times a day. Some doctors recommend checking each time insulin is taken, and at bedtime. Others suggest at least two checks a day, one of them upon arising. One day a week, check before every meal and at bedtime. Whatever the recommendation, many people on the intensive program want to check three to four times a day because the feedback is so valuable.

Step 9: Assess your progress and determine what (if anything) is needed to further improve control.

You may have made great progress, and most of your levels are within your target range. Or perhaps you have made significant improvements, but are still higher than you would like. It's possible that your checks show little improvement, even though you have followed every step of the intensive program carefully. Your blood sugar level may vary greatly, with frequent lows. Possibly you have been struggling just to check regularly.

No matter what you have achieved at this point, it is time to pause and congratulate yourself. Even if you are still out of control and not doing everything you know is good for you, it is time to reward yourself. Whether you have much or little to accomplish, take time to define your progress, what you need to learn, what obstacles are holding you back, and what you can do to overcome them.

If you need to further improve your control, go through the following checklist and see what you still need to learn.

1. Do you understand your insulin regimen—what type of insulin you are supposed to take and when each of them peaks? If not, go over your plan again with your doctor.
2. Do you understand what causes your blood sugar to go up and down? If not, reread Chapters 8, 9, and 12.
3. Is your blood sugar checking accurate? If you haven't been instructed in the proper technique, ask your doctor

or diabetes educator to help you. Do you need a new meter?

4. Is your life filled with stress, or are you especially sensitive to stress? If so, read Chapter 12 and consider taking a stress management class.
5. Are you finding it difficult to stick to a scheduled meal and exercise plan? If so, read pages 117–148.
6. Do you understand and follow your meal plan? Do you like it? If not, meet with the dietitian and get what you need.
7. Are you physically active every day or every other day? If not, start with a walking program (see page 145).
8. Do you notice any signs of nighttime low blood sugar? Have you checked your blood sugar during the night (around 2:00 or 3:00 a.m.) to be sure you are not having lows?
9. Are there any irregularities or imbalances in your endocrine hormones other than insulin? Your doctor can order tests to see if this is true.
10. Is any other physical condition affecting your control? Discuss this with your doctor.
11. Do you have strong doubts that optimal control is worth the effort it takes to achieve it? Do you believe that the intensive program intrudes on your life too much or creates too many inconveniences? Is your belief true?

    - ☐ Review page 56 on the benefits of the intensive program.
    - ☐ Review pages 234–235 on the complications of diabetes.
    - ☐ Try a support group to bolster your motivation.

12. Do you doubt yourself—either your ability to learn, or your worth as a person? Individual counseling may help.
13. Are you learning the intensive program at a time when the rest of your life is too demanding? It's possible that

problems with school, work, family, or relationships are competing with your need to manage your diabetes. If so, can you put any of the other challenges on hold? Or is it better to commit to the moderate program now?

14. Do you have enough support and guidance from your doctor and others?
15. Let your doctor and other health professionals know what you need. If your requests are legitimate and they are unwilling to meet them, consider changing doctors.
16. Have you enlisted the support of others with diabetes? (See Chapter 13.)
17. Is there anything else that could cause your difficulty?

Taking a Break

If you are tempted to quit because you're having difficulty gaining the level of control you want, you may need a short break from the intensive program. Step back and look at your whole situation. Even if your blood sugar checks are not yet on target, you might find that you have made progress by mastering some of the tasks of the intensive program. You haven't failed; there is just more to learn.

You may need to accept higher blood sugar levels while you work on your motivation, reduce your stress level, or handle other issues outside diabetes. You may also have physical conditions that make control more difficult to attain. You may need to find a doctor who is better informed or more sympathetic to your goals. If you want a referral to a different diabetes educator or diabetes education program, call the American Association of Diabetes Educators at 1-800-TEAM-UP-4 or the American Diabetes Association at 1-800-DIABETES.

If, after determining the reasons for your frustration, you decide to take a break from the intensive program, don't punish yourself. Make a commitment to reevaluate your decision at a scheduled date in the future. Write it on your calendar. Understand the reasons for your decision, and let them guide you to your next step in diabetes education. Follow the moderate program, and work on the issues that have prevented you from succeeding with the intensive program. (For a quick look at the differences between the moderate and intensive programs, see the chart on page 82.) If you discontinue the intensive program without blaming yourself, you will find it much easier to begin again later.

You may also decide, on the basis of this experience with the intensive program, that you do not want to manage diabetes at this level. Try to find a new diabetes educator; this sometimes makes all the difference.

Step 10: Maintain your motivation.

The intensive program becomes easier to manage once you know the basics. The glucose checking schedule is not as demanding, you can be flexible in lifestyle and still maintain good control, and you have a new set of habits that help you live well with diabetes. Your program is easier, and your life runs more smoothly because of it. You have assumed a position of responsibility, one calling for daily awareness and decision making. Congratulate yourself daily for this.

The immediate rewards of following the intensive program reinforce your motivation. When you have quick feedback regarding your blood sugar levels and have the ability to do something about them, you enjoy a sense of power and control. This emotional benefit is reinforced by the feeling of physical well-being that accompanies optimal control. Don't take these improvements for granted. Remember that you have worked hard to achieve them and that you will continue to enjoy them by maintaining your program.

You can also use the long-term benefits of optimal control as motivation to stick with your program. You are increasing your chances of living a long and healthful life. You are maintaining a body that functions like that of someone without diabetes. If you have children, you are more likely to be an active parent throughout their childhood. If you are a woman who wants to become pregnant, you can be more assured of having a safe pregnancy and a healthy baby. Periodically, review why you want to live well, and keep in mind how the intensive program will help you get what you want in life.

Contact with others following the same program can also reinforce your motivation. Participation in a support group, or having friends with diabetes you can talk to when you need understanding and encouragement, helps in a unique way. You are talking with people who know what you are dealing with. You can get practical tips from experienced people, and you will soon be giving advice to beginners. It is easier to stay involved with quality self-care when you know you are not alone.

Take a brief vacation from intensive management as a way of relieving any sense of burden. With the skills you have learned in varying insulin, food intake, and exercise, you can relax for a day or two and not end up with severely elevated blood sugar levels. (When doing this, don't create conditions that can cause severe low blood sugar reactions, such as taking too much rapid-acting insulin, eating late meals, or eating too much quickly-absorbed carbohydrate.) It is much easier to continue with the intensive program if you do not think of it as a straightjacket and any departure as cheating. Living well includes brief periods of relaxed control as part of the program.

Step 11: Celebrate!

When you finish learning the intensive program, you understand the most demanding body of information medicine has to offer its patients. Celebrate your accomplishment; let your family and friends know what it means to you. After all, most of what you are doing to live well with diabetes would also help them live more healthful lives. Share the joy of reaching your goal; it will help you to continue your new level of self-care. You can take this task literally and have a party or a special dinner to announce your "graduation." It can be as subtle or as exuberant as you want.

If you have a reward system, now is the time to collect whatever prize you contracted for. Even if you haven't been working with this idea in mind, you might want to give yourself something. It might be an experience you have been postponing, a relationship you have not felt ready for, or even time alone, away from all other demands. You will know what is right for you.

You will also know that you still need to learn about diabetes. Mastering the intensive program does not mean that you have finished your diabetes education. Reread the other chapters of this book to pick up concepts you may have missed before. See Appendix 1 for other sources of information. Fortunately, you are engaged in a lifelong learning process, as there will always be new research, different techniques for diabetes care, and technology breakthroughs to help you feel even better.

CHAPTER

7

If You'd Rather Not Choose a Program

If you find yourself not wanting to choose any wellness program—in fact, not taking care of your diabetes very well at all—please reconsider. Give yourself the gift of health. The power to feel better can be yours. If you believe that you control your diabetes management, you are more likely to realize other self-care choices are possible. You will live longer, feel better, and minimize your chances of complications if you start taking care of yourself now.

> It sure would have helped if someone had told me I was choosing to be out of control. I never saw that I was the one who went on binges or "forgot" my shot and that's why my blood sugar was out of whack. It seemed like it just happened, like somebody else was doing it to me. But I was really in control all along.
>
> —Joe, 29

Is any of the following true for you?

- Your life is in turmoil or filled with external demands.
- You value maintaining your current lifestyle over preventing future problems.

- You feel rebellious or unwilling or unable to change.
- You have a poor self-image and think you can't do any better.
- You are broke and can't afford the necessary supplies for other programs, or you don't want to spend money on them.
- You don't believe complications are going to happen to you.

If some of these descriptions fit you, you may want to try some of the ideas below.

1. **If your life is filled with external demands or is in turmoil,** set aside some minimum amount of time for learning to manage your diabetes more effectively. As little as 10–20 minutes a day can be a good beginning. The important thing is to make a commitment in spite of a challenging schedule or an overwhelming set of problems. Once you have begun, it may be easier for you to give diabetes care a higher priority and give more time to it. You may find that some of those other tasks can be scaled down or put on hold for a while. If not, you will at least learn information and skills vital to your well being. You also are likely to find that you feel better physically. This can give you more strength to deal with your other life demands.

2. **If you have chosen to ignore your diabetes because you tend to live for the moment,** valuing present pleasures over future risks, you may be surprised. Many people following more intensive programs report no shortage of enjoyable experiences. For them, greater control gives them greater freedom. Regular blood glucose testing and the ability to adjust insulin, food, and exercise allow great flexibility in lifestyle, at a relatively small sacrifice of time.

This freedom in living carries with it less anxiety about the future. People who are actively controlling diabetes are doing the best they can to reduce the risk of complications later in life. You will be amazed at how much better you feel physically when your blood sugar levels are close to normal.

You will find it useful to review the main pleasures in your life and ask yourself how they can be reconciled with improved diabetes care. There are relatively few absolute contradictions, so long as you are not attached to excess itself as a pleasure. It might help you to talk with others who are following more intensive programs and have found ways to respect the pleasure principle.

Although you may feel set in your habits, you should remember that human beings are very adaptable. You can probably think of changes that have occurred in your own life that at first seemed very negative but soon proved to be definite improvements.

3. **If you feel rebellious or unwilling or unable to change,** you may want to work on issues of power. Diabetes programs are easier to follow if you feel you are in charge, not the doctor. You are the one who ultimately decides what you will or will not do, no matter what your doctor says. If you see doctors as authorities who give orders, and you then act against their advice, your rebellion is hardly freedom. If you feel weak and unable to do what your doctor says, this too is a form of rebellion, though more subtle. Either way, you lose.

Real freedom and power come from consciously deciding what you will do in each situation you face. Even if your doctor does tend to give commands, hear them as intelligent advice. Make conscious decisions about what you will or will not do and give yourself room to make new decisions later.

4. **If you feel you don't deserve first-class care,** you may need to work on developing a more positive self-image. Unfortunately, negative beliefs about yourself tend to produce behavior that reinforces them. Escape from this cycle can take place through changes in the beliefs themselves or in the behavior. A counselor can help you, but many people have made changes at this level by themselves. The key is to believe that you deserve health.

5. **If you lack the money for home blood glucose testing or other diabetes care supplies,** seek help from your doctor, diabetes educator, or dietitian. They can help you search for community resources that may provide you with essential supplies. Many health insurance companies now cover testing supplies and equipment, as well as diabetes education. Most states have also passed laws requiring health insurance companies to pay for necessary equipment, supplies, and education. Also, search the Internet for discount mail order supply houses offering significant savings.

6. **Unfortunately, serious complications of diabetes will result** if you have high blood sugar levels over time. Believe it. You can work to prevent them—but not without paying attention to your blood sugar levels.

6 Steps to Start Now

If you are not taking care of your diabetes at all, we urge you to start by learning the following six steps.

Step 1: Learn what you need to know to stay alive.

Know about low blood sugar and how to treat it (see Chapter 10). Know the signs of diabetic ketoacidosis (diabetic coma; see page 155). Know about your risk of developing complications (see Chapter 11). Treat any infection promptly. See your doctor often.

Step 2: Learn to do home blood glucose checks.

Ask your doctor or diabetes educator to teach you, or take a class. As few as two blood sugar checks a week have proven effective in helping people with diabetes improve their metabolic control. Keep the test strips available so you can easily check when you want to know how changes in food, activity, or stress have affected your blood sugar levels. If you think your blood sugar has become high, check it and validate your perception. When you become ill, blood glucose checks make it much easier to prevent blood sugar levels from skyrocketing. This can promote quick recovery.

Also learn how to test your urine for ketones. This test is especially important because it indicates when your control is significantly off due to physical illness, emotional stress, or very high blood sugar levels.

Step 3: Take diabetes pills and/or one or two insulin shots daily.

If you have type 1, taking more injections or using the insulin pump are not recommended without more blood sugar checks. If you have type 2, take the prescribed medications and shots on a schedule outlined by your doctor.

Step 4: Eat healthfully and in moderation.

Learn how to increase the pleasure of eating without increasing the calorie and fat content of your snacks and meals. If you overeat, binge eat, and ignore your meal plan, you might find Chapter 8 helpful. It contains tips on ways to enjoy food while eating more healthfully.

Step 5: Observe great caution in adjusting insulin dosage.

Be cautious in adjusting insulin dosage to compensate for changes in food intake and activity level. You need the feedback of regular blood sugar checks to do this safely. If your blood sugar is high because you are ill, consult with your doctor on any changes in the amount of insulin you take. Always consult your doctor before making any changes in your medication if you have type 2 diabetes.

Step 6: Make a commitment to continue diabetes learning, maintain your motivation, and review obstacles to improved control.

Explore what commitment you are prepared to make to continue learning about diabetes self-care. Determine the aspects of diabetes management that you are willing to work on. By proceeding this way, you are likely to learn more quickly.

Scan the sections of the moderate and intensive regimens to see if you are interested in learning about them. Look again through the Table of Contents and find what you are now willing to learn about. A conversation with your physician or diabetes educator might help you define your next goals.

Our hope is that you begin the moderate program as soon as you can, so that you can live a long and healthy life.

PART THREE

The Keys to Success

CHAPTER 8

Eating Well

"Tell me what you eat, and I shall tell you what you are," wrote Brillat-Savarin in 1825. Food and eating are an inextricable part of our culture and our daily lives. We use eating to sustain ourselves, reward ourselves, and comfort ourselves. We center social occasions and family gatherings around food. When other things in our life may be out of our control, we count on being able to eat what we want, no matter the cost.

I couldn't stand it when my doctor told me I had diabetes. All I could think about was having to give up everything I loved to eat. I just didn't want to do that. I didn't care how sick I got, really. I just wanted to be able to eat what I wanted to eat. It seemed like such a basic right.

—Sally, 52

All of us know some foods are healthier than others. All of us know eating too much will make us fat. Most of us are very conscious of how particular foods affect how we feel. We know we should eat less animal fat, less sugar, more fiber. But why are so many of us—with and without diabetes—unwilling to stick to a healthy meal plan?

Two reasons: we've trained our taste buds to think high-fat, high-sugar foods taste better. And we've attached emotional meanings to particular foods or to eating in general. Is any of the following true for you?

- I think I have the right to eat whatever I want.
- After all I do every day, I *deserve* to eat whatever I want.
- I don't get much else out of life, so I should be able to enjoy my food.
- When I eat ________ (some unhealthy food), I feel __________ (in some way better: loved, comforted, or satisfied).
- I don't deserve to feel healthy.
- I don't care if I am healthy.

Feelings like these will always keep you from sticking to a healthy meal plan. It doesn't matter how many times you visit your dietitian or sit down to plan healthy meals.

Buying In (and What's Changed)

To succeed at a healthy meal plan, you need to do three things:

- Design a meal plan with a dietitian that has foods in it you already like.
- Gradually start eating healthier foods that will soon—believe it or not—taste better to you than junky foods.
- Realize when you are eating emotionally, and find other ways to deal with those emotions.

The single hardest thing for most people with diabetes to do is change the way they eat. Being unwilling or unable to stick to a meal plan is the cause of most high blood sugar levels, which in turn cause diabetic complications. Many people who've just been diagnosed give up right at the point their doctor says, "you'll need to lose some weight." Most people feel depressed, discouraged, and angry about having to give up their favorite foods.

The first thing you need to realize is this: **there is no more "diabetic diet," and you don't have to give up your favorite foods**. You just have to eat them in moderation. Having diabetes doesn't mean the end of life as you know it, food-wise. It used to. We used to think you couldn't eat sugar or sweets if you had diabetes. This was very depressing to a lot of people. Many people with diabetes still think this, feel sorry for themselves, and don't eat well.

We now know that **your meal plan is the same as that of any healthy person without diabetes.** It provides healthy sources of protein, fat, and carbohydrate in the right quantities. It's not having diabetes that makes eating this way necessary. It's being human. We all have to eat the right quantities of the right foods in order to be healthy.

You are going to feel worse sooner than people without diabetes if you don't eat right, sure. But we'll all die from unhealthy eating eventually.

What about your doctor's comment that you're going to have to lose weight? Do you know why (other than the obvious)? If you are overweight, losing weight is one of the single greatest steps you can take to bring your diabetes under control. Often people with type 2 who have to go on meds or insulin can reduce or completely eliminate them just by losing weight.

That's because having too much fat, especially on the upper body, decreases your body's ability to use insulin. This is called insulin resistance. Being overweight also strains your pancreas, and it has a harder time making the insulin your body needs. So, by getting rid of excess body fat, you can improve your sensitivity to insulin. This will help you get your diabetes under much better control.

Setting up a healthy weight loss plan is not much different than a healthy eating plan for someone who doesn't need to lose weight. You'll need to eat fewer calories than you're used to. You still want to eat a great variety of foods and include lots of vegetables, grains, and fruits. But you won't necessarily have to eat less food. One simple—and healthy—way to lose weight is to cut down on the fat in your meal plan. And—of course—you have to move around a little. Yes, physical activity (see Chapter 9). Your dietitian will help you devise a weight loss plan with the right amount of calories, fat, and carb for you.

How to Do It (and Stick to It)

Once you understand the total amount of calories, fat, and carb grams you need, you can mix and match your foods just like anyone else. So see your dietitian and talk about how you currently eat. (To find a dietitian, ask your doctor, or call 1-800-366-1655 or 1-800-TEAMUP4). Your dietitian should ask you many questions about when, what, and why you're eating certain things. Some of the questions might be:

- What are your favorite foods?
- Which foods do you dislike?
- When are you hungriest?
- What do you snack on? When do you snack?
- Do you exercise?
- What foods do you want to see on your meal plan all the time? Some of the time?
- Which foods do you eat too much of?
- When do you find yourself overeating?

You can try the questionnaire on the next page to start thinking about your eating habits.

My Eating Habits

1. My current weight is: ______________.

2. My target weight is: ______________.

3. I think of food as:

____

4. My favorite foods are:

____

____

____

____

____

5. I can't stand to eat:

____

____

____

6. I would like to change the following about my eating habits:

____

____

____

7. My current physical activities are:

____

____

8. I would like to change the following about my physical activities:

____

____

9. I find myself eating when I am:

- hungry
- tired
- lonely
- depressed
- sad
- irritated
- bored
- happy

10. The foods I eat at these times are:

____

____

11. Instead of eating at these times, I could:

____

____

Your dietitian may ask you to keep a food diary for a week to record how much food you're actually eating (see the sample on pages 124–125). For a solid week, write down everything you eat. Don't leave out anything. You want to get an honest assessment of what (and why) you're eating. Make sure you describe each food, the serving size, and how you were feeling before and after you ate it.

Writing down everything you eat throughout the day is sometimes a shock. A food diary is very useful, though, because it can reveal times you're eating because of something you're feeling. Your dietitian should help you realize any emotional eating you may be doing, and should be able to offer suggestions if this is a problem for you. After finding out your likes, dislikes, and exercise level, your dietitian will ask you about any meds or insulin you're on and when you take them.

You'll decide on a target weight and find out how many calories you need to meet that target. A reasonable weight loss rate is one or two pounds a week. Since each pound equals 3,500 calories, you will have to reduce your total food intake by at least 500 calories a day. So if you are used to eating

3,000 calories a day, you should eat 2,500 each day to lose one pound a week, or 2,000 calories per day to lose two pounds each week. Over 85% of people with type 2 diabetes are overweight when diagnosed. Losing just 10 or 20 pounds can make your body more responsive to the insulin it produces. You may be able to lower your medication dose or stay off insulin. Losing weight helps lower your blood lipids and blood pressure. And you already know how much better you'd feel.

Choose a Meal Planning Method

After choosing a target weight, you'll learn to plan your meals with the right amount of calories, fat, and carbohydrate for you using one or a combination of the following meal plan systems.

Using Exchanges

The Exchange System was developed to help you balance your food needs with your food preferences. Foods that are alike are in the same group. All the foods in the group have about the same amount of carbohydrate, protein, fat, and calories. That means you can trade foods in the same group back and forth to vary your plan. You can pick the foods you like best to eat as long as they're in the same group. The groups are Meat and Meat Substitutes, Starch, Vegetables, Milk, Fat, Fruit, Other Carbohydrates (that's a good one; lots of tasty desserts), and one called Free (things like low-sugar jam, fat-free salad dressing, and salsa, all in the right quantities). Bread, cereals, pasta, beans, and starchy vegetables are starches. Meat is divided into very lean, lean, medium fat, and high fat.

For example, if you wanted to have a special breakfast out with your friends, you could have 2 meat exchanges, 1 fat exchange, 2 starch exchanges, 1 vegetable exchange, and

Food Diary

Day Time	Food Eaten	Blood Sugar

Emotional Feelings		Physical Feelings	
Before	After	Before	After

1 fruit exchange. That would translate into 1/2 cup tomato juice, 1 scrambled egg, 1 ounce ham, 1/3 cup hash browns, 1 muffin, and 1 cup melon cubes. Your dietitian will help you plan how much of each category you need at each regular meal and snack and how to plan for parties and holidays. You'll need the book *Exchange Lists for Meal Planning*, available from the American Diabetes Association, if you're using this system.

Carb Counting

We found out an incredible thing recently that is going to greatly improve your life with diabetes. It turns out that a baked potato will raise your blood sugar as high as a brownie. That means that a baked potato is not automatically "good" and a brownie "bad." They're both forms of carbohydrate. And any carbohydrate will raise your blood sugar level.

The trick is to find out the number of grams of carb in each food, then trade the carb grams around depending on how many you need to keep your blood sugar stable. That's how people with diabetes now eat brownies! They account for the total carb in their meal plan. They don't eat brownies at every meal . . . but no one does. They eat whatever they like in moderation and account for the total carb (and calories and fat) in their meal plan.

How do you count carb? First, find out how many grams (g) of carb are in the foods you eat. How do you do that? You buy a book that tells you, or you read food labels.

- Each starch, fruit, milk, starchy vegetable (like corn, peas, and potatoes), and other carbohydrate exchange has 15 g carb. A vegetable serving has about 5 g carb (another reason to eat more veggies). You don't count carb in meat or fat because there isn't any.
- Nutrition Facts on a food label tell you grams of carb as Total Carbohydrate. (Ignore the grams of sugar—they're

part of the Total Carb.)

- Bonus: if you eat 5 or more grams of fiber (part of Total Carb), subtract that number from your carb grams for the meal. (This is another benefit of high-fiber foods such as whole grains, fruits, and vegetables!) Fiber slows down the rise in blood sugar, too.
- Double-check the serving size on the label. If you're actually eating two servings, you're getting twice as much carb as is on the label.
- For the thousands of foods without a label, buy (or check out at the library) books listing carb counts. New cookbooks have this information, too.

Nutrition Facts

Serving Size 1 cup (228g)
Servings Per Container 2

Amount Per Serving

Calories 260 Calories from Fat 120

	% Daily Value*
Total Fat 13g	**20%**
Saturated Fat 5g	**25%**
Cholesterol 30mg	**10%**
Sodium 660mg	**28%**
Total Carbohydrate 31g	**10%**
Dietary Fiber 0g	**0%**
Sugars 5g	
Protein 5g	

Vitamin A 4% • Vitamin C 2%
Calcium 15% • Iron 4%

* Percent Daily Values are based on a 2,000 calorie diet. Your daily values may be higher or lower depending on your calorie needs:

	Calories:	2,000	2,500
Total Fat	Less than	65g	80g
Sat Fat	Less than	20g	25g
Cholesterol	Less than	300mg	300mg
Sodium	Less than	2,400mg	2,400mg
Total Carbohydrate		300g	375g
Dietary Fiber		25g	30g

Calories per gram:
Fat 9 • Carbohydrate 4 • Protein 4

Reading labels may not sound like a lot of fun at first, but when you realize reading food labels is your key to making food *choices*, it's not so bad. You want to make wise food choices—more vegetables than dessert, more fresh foods than processed ones. Why? Because whole grains and vegetables give you the vitamins, minerals, and fiber you need. They're premium fuel for your body.

Next, find out how much carb to eat. For most adults, it's 4–5 carb exchanges at each meal, or 60–75 g carb. It's better to eat some carb at each meal instead of all at one meal (this will send your blood sugar sky high!). Your goal is to eat about the same amount of carb at the same meal each day, so your blood sugar levels fall into a predictable pattern.

The best way to determine how different foods affect you is to try them and measure their effect on your blood sugar one or two hours after you've eaten. This feedback helps you know the types and amounts of food that are appropriate for you. And it helps you change your meal plan when your tests are high.

If you take insulin before meals, you can adjust the amount of insulin you take based on how much carb you expect to eat. The amount of insulin you need to process carb varies from person to person. That's why keeping good records of food intake and blood sugar level is so important. As you fine-tune your diabetes care, you will learn to adjust for many different eating situations. That's freedom.

Eat in Moderation

This is hard for almost everyone. Here are some tips that may help.

- **Start to exercise.** When you feel like eating, exercise instead. This really works to control food cravings. If you feel like eating at night in front of the TV, buy an exercise machine and get on it.

- **Know correct portion sizes.** Healthy portion sizes are, sadly, much smaller than what we're used to in our culture. The right amount of protein to eat at a meal is the size of the palm of your hand. One serving of mashed potatoes is 1/2 cup. A serving of rice is 1/3 cup. It's unbelievable, but true.

Again, adjust to this slowly. You don't want to set up any feelings of deprivation and make yourself so mad you quit eating right. Gradually start reducing your serving sizes and find other ways to feel satisfied. You can:

- have soup or salad before your main meal.
- add more fiber-rich foods to your meal that fill you up.
- eat more slowly (it takes 20 minutes to feel full).
- stop eating before you feel full.
- use smaller plates, bowls, and glasses.
- avoid putting serving bowls on the table (fill your plate once in the kitchen and don't go back for more).
- drink liquids with your meals to feel full.

- **Become a taster.** Eat just a bite or two of an unexpected treat. If you want more, figure out how to accommodate it in your meal plan.

- **Eliminate guilt.** Instead, plan. You can eat these foods. You just have to figure out how!

- **Figure out what your trigger foods are** (foods that you tend to overeat), and only eat them on social occasions with friends. Share any sweet desserts. Declare your portion intentions at the beginning. Say, "I'm going to eat three bites of this pie and that's it." Then do it. Don't keep trigger foods in your house.

- **Plan for challenges,** such as parties or times when you're bored or depressed. Tell someone in advance what you intend to eat. Then have that person eat with you or call them after the party. If you know you have to report in to someone, it can help you stay motivated.

- **Solve your meal plan problems.** If you don't like it or can't stick to it, get back to the dietitian and make some changes. If you have to eat later than usual, have a small snack or change the timing of your insulin dose. Always carry healthy snacks with you and know when to use them. During holidays, if food is going to be out all day and you're not on insulin, try dividing your total daily food into snack-size meals. Then you can spread the food out throughout the day without going over your total.

- **Get interested in what else life has to offer.** Food can't be your reward or your comfort anymore. You have to find other ways of making yourself happy. This is hard. Make a list of everything you like to do. Add some things you always wanted to try but never had the time or energy for. Talk to your friends and family about fun things you can do together. Reach for a book, the phone, or a child when your food cravings start. Write a letter. Go for a walk. After awhile, these activities will feel more natural to you than eating.

- **Don't waste time on guilt.** If you overeat one day, get right back on your meal plan the next. Don't use the previous day as an excuse to really blow it. Instead, love yourself enough to see that day as a learning opportunity, and try again.

- **Join a support group or see a counselor.** Don't hesitate to find other ways to help yourself. Eating right and losing weight are issues almost everyone struggles with. Find out what helped other people. You are not alone in this!

Cooking Tips

You can also make a lot of improvements in your cooking techniques. You've heard all these things before. But this time, as you go through the list, start actually implementing each change. You don't have to do everything at once. It takes time for your taste buds to readjust. Just try one or two changes until they become habits. Then try another one or two changes. In a few months, you'll be cooking in a whole new way . . . and you'll be liking it.

- ☐ Use low-fat or fat-free versions of things: milk, cheese, salad dressings, yogurt, soups, meat, ice cream. But watch out: sometimes they have more calories or carb than the regular version.
- ☐ Broil or bake foods instead of frying or sautéing them. Use nonstick cookware.
- ☐ Buy lean cuts of meat. Trim visible fat before cooking. Avoid eating poultry skin.
- ☐ Use cooking sprays instead of oil. If you use oil, try olive or canola.
- ☐ Use artificial sweeteners in moderation instead of sugar, and diet drinks instead of full-sugar varieties (you probably already do this).
- ☐ Use fresh herbs, lemon juice, flavored vinegars, garlic, onion, or salt substitute blends instead of extra salt.
- ☐ Eat more fiber (found in vegetables, grains, beans, and fruit).
- ☐ Buy low-fat or low-calorie frozen meals. These have portion control built right in.
- ☐ Eat more fresh fruit and cut down on fruit juices (according to your carb requirements). Whole fruit has more fiber than juice.
- ☐ If you eat out in restaurants, select lower-fat choices. Even fast-food restaurants have low-fat choices now.

Experiment with your favorite recipes to see how the flavor changes when you use less fat. Use yogurt or fruit purees to give texture to baked goods. Use fat-free evaporated milk to make things rich and creamy. Try recipes from diabetes cookbooks and use those same techniques and ingredients in your favorite recipes.

There are many great low-carb cookbooks out now. Try some new recipes and see if you like them. If the carb count of your favorite recipe is too high, eat a smaller serving. A smaller piece of your favorite pie may satisfy you more than a large piece of the low-fat or low-carb version.

Edward Espe Brown, a Zen priest, poet, chef, and cookbook writer, wrote in 1991 that "food is not just food, something 'out there;' food is our body, the body of the world, the way the body of the world becomes our body. . . Eating with awareness, we know that life is delicious. . . . We join again the ageless dance of life—and rejoice." Find life, and your meal plan, delicious again.

CHAPTER

9

Enjoying Physical Activity

> One of the good things about diabetes is that it makes a virtue out of enjoying myself physically. The little doctor in the back of my head smiles when I go dancing or swimming, even when I make love. My prescription includes having fun!
>
> **—Linda, 47**

Everybody knows the benefits of staying fit. Exercise decreases the risk of heart disease, lowers high blood pressure, improves physical fitness and general health, reduces anxiety and depression, and enhances your sense of well being. As a person with diabetes, you enjoy an extra bonus: being active helps you control blood sugar levels and it lessens the risk of some complications.

How does exercise help you manage diabetes?

- Physical activity lowers your blood sugar by burning it as fuel. You can use exercise to return blood glucose levels to normal when tests are high (if test levels are not higher than about 300 mg/dl.

- Steady exercise for more than 20 minutes enables your muscles to store glucose, further lowering blood sugar levels after you've stopped exercising. Your body uses this store when your blood sugar levels become too low. When you exercise regularly, your blood sugar levels will be more stable.
- Consistent physical activity that is moderate or strenuous increases a cell's ability to use insulin. This lowers your necessary insulin dose.
- Exercise builds physical fitness, strengthening the heart, circulatory system, lungs, and muscles. This reduces the risk of cardiovascular complications.
- Exercise is a key to losing or controlling weight, and is as important as your meal plan in doing so.
- You can neutralize the effects of emotional stress with physical activity.
- Exercising makes you feel good!

Regular physical activity is a key ingredient of your diabetes wellness program, especially if you want optimal control. Exercise reduces your body's overall insulin requirement, compensates for blood sugar highs, and gives you greater balance in blood sugar levels (once you have adapted to exercising). The cardiovascular benefits are especially important to you because, as a person with diabetes, you have a higher risk of heart and circulatory difficulties. So, in addition to improving your metabolic control, a consistent exercise program can help prevent a heart attack and improve your circulation.

The benefits of exercise also exist at an emotional level. The increased flow of blood and oxygen to the cells and the hormonal shifts that occur when we are physically active lift our spirits. Counteract a stressful day at work with a brisk walk or game of tennis. Lighten your mild depression with an hour of working in the garden or riding a bike. When we are active, we have fewer mood swings and it is much easier to handle difficult problems.

How does all of this magic occur? As soon as we begin exercising, our muscles demand more energy. Blood flow to the muscles increases and more oxygen and glucose move into the muscle cells. Blood supply to the skin also increases, so the heat generated can be radiated out of the body. As an exercise session progresses, the liver releases additional glucose to fuel the muscles. Fats are also burned to provide further energy.

After you stop exercising, the effects continue to accumulate if you have been playing or working at a moderate to strenuous level. The liver and muscles need to restore their supply of glucose, and they draw it from the bloodstream when you are resting. This process can go on for several hours following strenuous activity. This is why low blood sugar reactions sometimes occur long after you've stopped exercising.

Exercise helps you lose weight by burning fat and turning glucose into muscle instead of more fat. Combining exercise with the proper meal plan allows a degree of weight control that cannot be obtained by diet alone. In fact, some weight-control programs now recommend at least one week of exercise before you begin dieting; the increase in activity level apparently makes appetite control easier.

The power of exercise to relieve stress symptoms is easy to explain: at the most basic level, the stress response is designed to prepare us to act physically. When stressed, we are ready for "fight or flight," so the most natural way to deal with stress is to move vigorously in order to use the hormones and glucose generated by it. This also enables us to release the physical tension that usually accompanies stress, assuming that the exercise includes a relaxed warm-up period.

Short-term benefits follow any period of increased physical activity. But when you continue activity long enough to raise your pulse to the target range for your age, for 15–20 minutes or more a day, you achieve what is called "the training effect" (see page 141). If you do this regularly for a few weeks, you begin to enjoy the long-term benefits of exercise.

A consistent program of physical training gives you greater sensitivity to insulin (less insulin resistance), usually allowing a significant decrease in insulin dosage or modification of your medication dosage if you have type 2 diabetes. Your muscles store more glucose, which is readily available to balance low blood sugar. Reactions may become less severe as a result. Your body performs better, your lungs breathe deeper, your heart is stronger, and you feel better. You are living well!

Before you begin your program of physical activity, figure out what your activity level is by answering the following questions.

Your Activity Profile

1. My typical day includes

_____ hours of sleep (7–8 hours recommended)

_____ hours of low activity (riding in or driving a car, reading, desk work, watching television, eating, talking while sitting or standing)

_____ hours of moderate activity (walking, gardening, mopping, light labor; sports such as golf, bowling, or easy swimming)

_____ hours of vigorous activity (running, bicycling, tennis, or basketball; moderate to heavy labor such as digging or carrying heavy objects)

2. At least _____ times a week I increase this to

_____ hours of moderate activity

_____ hours of vigorous activity

_____ This increase of activity happens only on weekends.

_____ This activity is distributed through the week.

_____ Although I am usually sedentary, I have occasional bursts of heavy physical activity.

3. _____ I do some form of stretching or warm up before physical activity.
_____ I stretch to cool down after exercise.

4. The physical activities I enjoy most are:
____

Activities I would like to learn are:
____

5. I have the following conditions, which need to be considered in designing my activity program:
_____ Difficulty recognizing the signs of low blood sugar
_____ Heart disease
_____ High blood pressure
_____ Poor circulation
_____ Retinopathy
_____ Neuropathy (especially if it involves decreased sensation in the feet)
_____ Fatigue
_____ Back pain (or other muscular or joint discomfort)
_____ Foot problems
_____ Other:___________________________________

(If you checked any of the above, discuss exercise with your physician. You may need tests to determine the level of activity advisable.)

6. I see the following obstacles to exercising:
_____ I don't feel I have enough time for it.
_____ I'm afraid I'll have too many reactions.
_____ I feel clumsy and uncomfortable with my body.
_____ I'm bored by physical activities; I prefer using my mind.
_____ I don't enjoy physical activity; it's a burden.

_____ I'd rather do other things.
_____ I don't have much energy.
_____ Other:_______________________________

7. I could overcome these obstacles to exercise by:
____

8. I would like to increase my level of activity by:
____

9. I would like to begin:
_____ Today
_____ This week
_____ This month

Beginning Your Activity Program

Without fail, wear a diabetes I.D. bracelet or necklace and inform any gym personnel, coaches, or fellow participants that you have diabetes and may need sugar in case of low blood sugar levels.

We advise you to begin any program of exercise gradually. You need to build strength, endurance, and flexibility so that you will be comfortable exercising. You also have to discover your particular balance between increased activity, insulin, and meal plan in order to avoid serious reactions. If you have diabetic complications or other physical conditions, you will need to proceed cautiously and with guidance from your doctor. If you are over 35, you should probably have a physical stress test to determine the level of exercise appropriate for you.

Choose activities that you enjoy. You should look forward to your exercise times as positive experiences, not as burdens or tasks. The following list contains several physical activities, ranked according to calories burned. If you have several favorite activities, you can choose among them to add variety and deal with changes in weather, mood, and physical state.

Although you may prefer to have a partner when exercising, you should also have activities you can do by yourself. If your only physical activity tends to be your work, either on the job or at home, you will benefit more if you find new ways to enjoy it. Focus on your bodily movements as though they were a dance or a sport. Don't be so fixed on the end product that you ignore your body.

Find something from the ideas below that you'd enjoy doing.

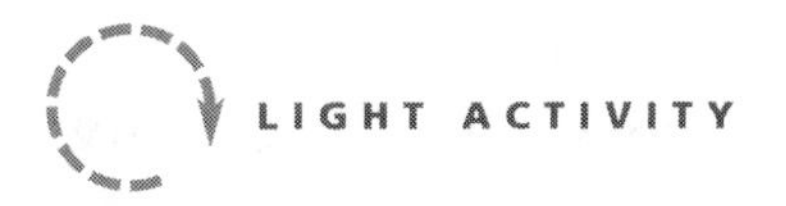

LIGHT ACTIVITY

Stretching
Slow walking
Light housekeeping
T'ai Chi
Yoga
Slow social dancing

MODERATE ACTIVITY

Moderate to fast walking
Tennis (doubles)
Stationary bicycle
Ice skating
Having sex
Volleyball
Bicycling
Calisthenics
Canoeing, kayaking, rowing
Fencing
Walking up stairs
Ballroom dancing
Gardening
Bowling
Swimming
Ping pong and badminton
Jogging
Jumping rope
Golf
Horseback riding
Square dancing or folk dancing
Aerobic dancing
Roller skating

VIGOROUS ACTIVITY

Digging and shoveling
Hiking
Tennis (singles)
Stair climbing
Bicycle racing
Racquetball
Ice skating
Squash and handball
Skiing (downhill and cross country)
Running
Chopping wood
Waterskiing
Basketball
Football
Moving furniture
Hill climbing
Soccer

You should always warm up before vigorous activity. More importantly, you should cool down afterwards. Stretching and warming muscles for five minutes and beginning exercise at a moderate pace allows your pulse and blood pressure to increase gradually. Cooling down with five or more minutes of mild activity allows your body to return to normal in the same manner. Neglecting to warm up or cool down can cause risky, abrupt shifts in pulse and blood pressure.

Although any activity helps you become more fit, you will receive the greatest benefit from exercise that requires a fairly steady level of exertion and movement (such as jogging, dancing, or swimming). Stop-and-start activities (such as tennis and volleyball) and static straining (weight lifting) do not build the same level of fitness in your cardiovascular system. However, many people enjoy strength training. Strength training uses special machines or hand weights to provide resistance that strengthens and tones your muscles as you go through a series of exercises. There are people to help you get started at health clubs, adult education classes, and senior centers. Again, it's best to get information and some instruction before you begin.

How Do You Know When You're Exercising Beyond Your Limit?

- If you become faint, dizzy, or nauseated, if you experience severe shortness of breath or tightness or pain in your chest, or if you lose control of your muscles, stop immediately and contact your doctor.
- If your pulse or breathing rate does not return to normal within three minutes of stopping exercise, you are probably pushing yourself too hard and need to adjust your level of exercise.
- If you are fatigued by moderate activity, and especially if you continue to feel exhausted in the hours following, you are doing more than your current level of fitness will support. Cut back the duration or intensity of exercise until you feel stronger. (If this tiredness begins abruptly, it may indicate that you are coming down with a cold or the flu.)
- Be sure that you get enough water during exercise. You need to drink water every 15–20 minutes during strenuous activity.

The Training Effect

The greatest benefits of exercise occur when you reach the training effect. This is achieved through sustained activity that raises your pulse to your target level for at least 20 minutes. If you do this at least three times a week (every other day), both your heart and metabolic system will function better.

However, recent studies have shown that even short periods of activity are beneficial, such as three short walks of 10 minutes each per day. Moderate walking at the rate of about one mile every 15 minutes is also helpful. Any activity is beneficial to your health, just as it is to lowering blood sugar levels.

You have a built-in meter right at your fingertips for measuring the effectiveness and safety of physical activity. Count the number of heartbeats you can feel in your wrist or neck (just above the collarbone toward the center of your throat) for 15 seconds and multiply by four. This is your pulse rate. Do this before, during, and immediately following exercise. The following table gives the meaning of different pulse rates in terms of exercise intensity.

Pulse Rate (beats per minute)	Degree of Exertion You Feel	Comments
60–80	Very light	Of little value as exercise
80–100	Light	Useful if condition is very poor
100–120	Moderate	Intensity just right
120–140	Somewhat hard	Useful if condition is very good
140–160	Very hard	Stop! (Unless you are an athlete in top condition)

Those of you reluctant to stop and measure your pulse can use the degree of exertion that feels right to you as your guide. If you are unable to carry on a conversation, you might be overexerting yourself. If you work in the moderate to somewhat hard range, you will probably be at the level you need.

Another indicator of your level of physical condition is the time it takes your pulse to return to its resting rate after exertion. Measure your pulse after you have been resting for 15 minutes. Move vigorously until your pulse is over 120, then rest and measure your pulse at one-minute intervals. If it takes more than three minutes to return to your resting rate, you are in poor physical condition and need to proceed cautiously with your exercise program. A more precise way of assessing your condition is to undergo an endurance or stress test at your doctor's office or at a local YMCA or YWCA.

If you have been fairly sedentary, you might find that even mild activity will bring your pulse up to a high level. Your body is at a low level of physical condition, and your heart has to work hard to handle any increase in activity. Your limits will gradually increase, so don't push yourself too hard. Twelve to 20 minutes a day at a pulse rate of 100 to 120 is a good beginning. (If you are over 60 and have not been very active, start with five minutes a day.) Stay at this level for a couple of weeks, and increase the duration and intensity of activity only when your endurance increases.

As you get in better condition, you will find that you are exerting yourself harder before you reach the same pulse rate as you did previously with less activity. The flight of stairs that left you breathless and your heart pounding a few weeks ago will be easy. If you don't experience improved endurance, be sure to discuss this with your physician.

As you experience progress in endurance and performance, you will be able to gradually increase your level of activity. If your doctor approves, you can increase the duration and intensity of exercise every two or three weeks until you are at your peak. For a younger person without compli-

Age	Recommended Pulse Rate	Pulse Rate If You Have Heart Disease (Don't Exceed)
20	130–170	150
30	124–162	143
40	117–153	137
45	114–149	134
50	111–145	131
55	107–140	128
60	104–136	120
65	101–132	113

cations, peak performance will allow a pulse rate of 140 to 160 beats per minute for sessions of 30–60 minutes. It can take up to six months to reach this level of conditioning, depending on where you start. If you are older, set a lower target pulse rate depending on your age, according to the table on page 143.

How Often Do You Need to Exercise?

Three workout sessions a week can be enough to build conditioning. If you have diabetes, you also benefit from the blood sugar lowering effects. Ideally, you should include physical activity in your schedule every day. This regularity helps you maintain consistent blood sugar levels. You can't always meet this ideal, but you can use your skill at varying the ingredients of your wellness program to deal with varying levels of activity. You can tailor your meal plan or insulin dosage to the kind of day you have in mind. A few more units of insulin or smaller meals will help maintain your balance on inactive days.

What If You Have an Active Job?

Your work may be vigorous enough to keep you physically fit without further exercise. It depends upon the degree of exertion and the variety of movements you use. If your pulse stays in the range of 100–140 for extended periods during the day, you are working at a level that satisfies conditioning requirements. However, if your pulse is usually below 100 when on the job, you might need to exercise. If your job keeps you moving in repetitive patterns, you might need limbering exercises to avoid sore muscles and maintain flexibility.

Stretching

If you are already active in a sports program, you know the value of stretching exercises. For the rest of us, it would be beneficial to begin stretching every day.

Muscles that aren't frequently used tend to shorten and tighten and become more prone to injury. To remain limber requires only 5–15 minutes of stretching each day. There are special aids available such as rubber bands and sticks that help you hold positions for the 15 seconds required to get the benefit of a stretch. You need to begin gradually if you haven't been working out or have limited mobility. This is supposed to feel good, so don't push yourself into pain.

Developing an Exercise Program

To establish exercise habits that will really last, follow these guidelines.

1. **Build on the physical activities you already enjoy doing.** Your exercise program may take several hours a week for the rest of your life. Start with activities you enjoy, and then learn those you've always wished you could do. Avoid boredom by using several different forms of exercise.

2. **If you feel short on time, do things simultaneously.** Socialize and exercise at the same time (friends don't always have to talk sitting down!); use the exercise bicycle or stair climber while watching television, reading, or listening to music; hold business discussions as you walk.

3. **If you are reluctant to exercise because you feel clumsy and awkward, begin by walking.** It's hard to look clumsy while walking, and you can use walking to develop your coordination. The key is to pay attention to your body as you walk. Focus on your feet, legs, hips, arms, back, and shoulders. Let go of any tightness you notice. Later, you can apply this same awareness to any form of motion. You are likely to find any awkwardness decreasing as you learn to be conscious of your body and release its tensions.

4. Keep a balance between developing more endurance and staying comfortable. You need time to strengthen your heart and muscles and to learn how to adjust diet and/or insulin to your new level of exercise. If you go too fast, pain or low blood sugar might discourage you from continuing. This is especially important if you are over 35, if you have any signs of heart trouble, or if other complications have started to develop.

5. If competitive activities make you anxious, avoid them. The stress they create for you will offset the benefits of the exercise. (Others may find the spirit of competition necessary to maintain motivation and avoid boredom.)

6. Learn how to change your meal plan and/or insulin dosage to prepare for increased physical activity. It is better to have a few high blood sugar tests from eating more than it is to risk serious reactions. Feedback from your tests will tell you how much is enough. Exercise beginning 30–60 minutes after a meal is least likely to cause reactions. If activity comes two or more hours after eating, you should have a snack before you start, unless blood sugar is over 150 mg/dl.

7. If you have a distaste for exercise because you are an "intellectual" type, use the inner-sports approach. Techniques such as visualization, affirmation, and meditation help many people understand the strong relationship between mind and body and reinforce motivation to exercise. Try listening to books on tape while exercising. Another possibility is to keep an exercise log and get interested in your progress.

8. If you are hesitant to exercise because of limiting physical conditions, ask your doctor for guidelines to ensure safety. You might consider joining a class specifically designed for people with physical limitations. Your YMCA, March of Dimes, local ADA chapter, or adult-education school may have a program taught by someone trained to help you exercise safely and monitor your special condition. Organizations for the visually handicapped may also be of help.

Exercise and Blood Sugar Levels

If you are on insulin, home blood glucose testing and knowledge of your insulin program will help you avoid insulin reactions. If you test your blood sugar before exercise, 10–15 minutes after you stop, and one hour after that, you will see how different types and amounts of activity affect you. (The 10–15-minute delay after exercising is necessary because sugar from the liver may temporarily raise blood sugar during vigorous activity.) You will have a rough idea of how much exercise it takes to lower high blood sugar levels and when you need extra food or reduced insulin to raise them.

If your blood sugar is under 120 mg/dl before moderate to heavy activity, be sure to eat food that is absorbed quickly (fruit juice or dried fruit, for example). By trial and error, you will discover how much you need to eat before a given amount of exercise to avoid low blood sugar. For insulin users, keep in mind when your insulin tends to peak. Eat food if you are exercising at that time or match your activity to the times when insulin levels are not so high. The ideal time for exercise is about one hour after a meal; blood sugar is at a peak and reactions are less likely to occur. If you wait two hours or more, you should consider having a snack before physical activity, unless your blood sugar is high.

For insulin users, exercising the site where you injected the insulin (such as the thigh or the arm) causes the insulin to work faster. This can be an advantage if you need to bring down a high blood sugar level, or a disadvantage if you are at a normal level to begin with. If the level is normal, you should avoid legs as an injection site before a hike, or your racquet arm before a tennis match.

When you exercise strenuously or over a long period (over an hour), your blood sugar will continue to decrease after you stop. The muscles and liver are replenishing their stores of glucose from your bloodstream. This process can continue for several hours after exercise. You may need a larger meal or extra snacks to avoid low blood sugar reactions in the hours following high levels or extended periods of exertion.

Once you have learned to adjust diet and insulin dose, it becomes easier to avoid reactions caused by exercise. In fact, the increased glucose storage means you will enjoy more stable blood sugar levels. When levels begin to fall, more glucose is available to bring them back to normal.

If you lead an active life, especially if you are able to follow a consistent exercise program, there is an added benefit; you sensitivity to insulin is increased. This means that exercise will lower your blood sugar more and insulin will be more effective. You might be able to decrease your insulin dose by a few units, or more if you were previously sedentary.

Ironically, though, the ability of exercise to reduce your blood sugar is diminished when your blood sugar levels are higher than 250 or 300 mg/dl, especially if ketones are present. When we need it most, the effect of exercise is reversed, and your blood sugar may climb even higher. If your blood sugar level is higher then 250 mg/dl, don't try to bring it down with exercise

Keep in mind the overall interaction between insulin or diabetes pills, food, and activity. You can vary any one or a combination of these factors to compensate for high blood sugar levels or changes in routine. This allows you a high degree of flexibility while maintaining good blood sugar control.

If you are ill, you should avoid all but the mildest activities. Your body needs energy to deal with the stress of the illness. Exercise only adds to this physical stress and may worsen your condition.

CHAPTER 10

Avoiding Hypoglycemia

> There's nothing that makes me feel more anxious than the idea that I may just lose it if I don't eat enough or if I jog too far. I've had one reaction I didn't wake up from and one where I got so confused I forgot I was looking for food. My son finally came home and had to tell me what to do. I don't ever want to go through that again!
>
> **—Jan, 35**

What bothers you most about having diabetes? Is it having to change your lifestyle? Worrying about complications? Or is it the fear of hypoglycemia (low blood sugar)? If we don't respond adequately to the early warning signs, we can find ourselves in embarrassing situations because of things we did in a less-than-coherent state. Very low blood sugar levels result in unclear thinking and emotional outbursts. And if blood sugar levels fall too far, we can lose consciousness. We could even find ourselves waking up in the hospital or in jail. Is it any wonder we feel bothered by this?

The Action of Reaction

When blood sugar falls below a certain level (usually around 60–70 mg/dl), our body signals a red alert. Under stress, our body releases hormones that cause a racing pulse, nervousness, and sweating. This is our involuntary (or autonomic) nervous system going to work.

The response is appropriate, because the situation is serious. If our blood sugar levels become too low, we lose consciousness—our brain and central nervous system need glucose to function properly. At this point, if levels stay too low for too long, we risk brain damage. One of the hormones released in a serious reaction is glucagon, which releases glucose stored in the liver and helps raise blood sugar levels.

Low blood sugar can be caused by:

- eating too little or too late
- extra exercise or strenuous activity
- too much insulin
- certain diabetes pills
- getting very angry or upset

Well-managed diabetes depends on balancing the different factors affecting blood sugar level. Reactions occur because food, exercise, insulin or diabetes pills, and stress levels are out of balance. As we learn to regulate these factors, we learn to avoid reactions. We discover how different activities affect blood sugar and how to adjust food intake or medication dosage to compensate for increased activity. We learn what kind of stress is likely to lower blood sugar for us and how to compensate.

Symptoms

The symptoms of low blood sugar vary by person and type of reaction. If you think you're having a reaction, test your blood. If your blood glucose is below 60–70 mg/dl, it's time to eat a snack that will be rapidly absorbed. Test often at first as you develop and sharpen awareness of the symptoms that signal the onset of a reaction for you.

Symptoms of low blood sugar include:

- lightheadedness
- dizziness
- shakiness
- sweating
- increase in heart rate
- hunger
- blurry vision
- "fuzzy" mind
- mental confusion
- emotional outbursts
- numbness and tingling in the lips, tongue, or fingers
- extreme anxiety
- loss of consciousness
- convulsions

This sequence isn't always the same. Sometimes a reaction will approach very quietly, especially if the decrease in blood sugar has been slow. The first sign may be confusion or irritability. A person can forget that he or she is looking for candy or become distracted in their search. (If it's a nocturnal reaction, the person may dream or imagine that the candy has been eaten.) In some cases, a person may even become angry or resistant if anyone else suggests eating something sweet. Anger and change of personality are signs often recognized by those close to us.

Some people with diabetes do not experience the typical reaction symptoms. Because of reduced production of the hormones that signal a reaction, blood sugar can fall very low without producing symptoms. If you are not experiencing the usual symptoms of a reaction, discuss this with your doctor or diabetes educator. This is called "hypoglycemic unawareness," and you need some help in dealing with it.

To a large extent, the symptoms of a reaction and those of other conditions overlap. Anxiety or fear can cause a quickened pulse, cold hands, and shaking. Too many cups of coffee can produce a nervousness like that of a reaction. The hot flashes of menopause or other hormonal changes can mimic hypoglycemia. And rapidly falling blood sugar levels can produce symptoms of a reaction long before blood sugar really is low.

Treating a reaction when your symptoms are actually caused by anxiety can result in high blood sugar levels. It is best to test your blood whenever possible to verify that glucose levels are too low. However, any time you are in doubt and cannot test, it is better to eat some rapidly absorbed carbohydrate than risk a severe reaction. If the symptoms begin to decrease, it's likely your blood sugar was too low.

Sometimes people have all the symptoms of a reaction but their blood sugar is normal or high. Usually they have had high blood sugar for a long time. If this is the case for you, discuss it with your doctor.

The effects of alcohol or other drugs can also mask the symptoms of hypoglycemia. Someone who becomes even moderately intoxicated or high may not notice a reaction until blood sugar levels are quite low. The need for caution is compounded by alcohol, because this drug lowers blood sugar when one has not eaten for some time. Alcohol also blocks the liver's ability to release glucose into the blood. If you're on insulin, a couple of drinks before dinner can cause a severe reaction that you may not discover until the process has already advanced. If you choose to drink or use other drugs, it is best to check your blood sugar level frequently and eat a moderate snack beforehand.

Marijuana affects blood sugar by breaking down glycogen, a form of sugar stored in the liver and other body tissue. The release of glycogen increases blood glucose levels. There is no doubt about marijuana's other effect: inducing the "munchies." This drug-induced hunger combined with weakened inhibitions wreaks havoc on your meal plan. As with alcohol, marijuana decreases the awareness of an insulin reaction until it is far advanced, because the sensations of being high mask the symptoms. The more powerful forms of marijuana carry the added risk of drug dependency.

If you are on insulin, watch out for low blood glucose levels when you are sleeping at night. This may be a prolonged insulin reaction that occurs during sleep as a result of too much insulin in the bloodstream. The symptoms are usually not strong enough to wake you, and blood sugar does not continue to go down. Your body will release more glucose in an effort to counteract the reaction, and you'll have high blood sugar and ketones in the morning. (This is different from typical nighttime insulin reactions in which you either wake up in a sweat or don't wake up until the medics administer glucose to you.)

Ask your doctor about reducing your nighttime insulin dose or using a different type.

Reactions and Optimal Control

If you are tightly controlling your blood sugar, smaller falls in blood sugar can cause reactions. You may have more reactions than people who manage diabetes with moderate control. Their blood sugar levels fall rapidly, and their symptoms are usually strong and easily recognized. With tighter control, a decrease in blood sugar of only 20–30 mg/dl can be enough to cause a reaction, and the change can take place very gradually.

As a result, your symptoms are often much subtler. Slight confusion or unclear vision could be the only signs that your blood sugar has dropped to 50–60 mg/dl. You need to heighten your awareness and not expect all reactions to sound a strong alarm. Check blood sugar levels often and learn what your subtle signals are.

Those gaining optimal control may find that normal blood sugar levels feel rather uncomfortable and trigger symptoms of hypoglycemia. This is especially true if earlier blood sugar levels were consistently high. This is a brief occurrence, usually lasting no more than a week or two. The symptoms fade after you adjust to a more normal metabolism.

Treatment

The treatment for low blood sugar is 10–15 grams of rapidly absorbed carbohydrate, such as fruit juice, hard candies, or a cookie. Try any of the choices below.

1/2	cup orange or apple juice	2	tsp. jam
6	oz. cola (not diet)	2	Tbsp. raisins
1	fig bar cookie	1/2	oz. caramel or peanut brittle
2	2-inch chocolate chip cookies	5	LifeSavers
1	Tbsp. granulated sugar or honey	1–3	glucose tablets

Always carry a couple of servings of these items with you, and keep some in your glove compartment, desk, or locker. A roll of LifeSavers is especially convenient and inconspicuous.

When you are dealing with very low blood sugar, the temptation to overcompensate can be powerful. (This is especially true in the middle of the night, when blood sugar can fall to very low levels before you wake up.) However, if you want to avoid leaps in blood sugar levels, you need to treat reactions in stages. First eat 10–15 grams of carbohydrate, wait 10–15 minutes, and then eat another 10–15 grams if your symptoms have not subsided.

The exception to this practice would be when you are experiencing a very severe reaction following strenuous exercise or a missed meal. At such a time, you may need to double the amount of sugar to bring blood glucose back to normal. Unless a reaction occurs within an hour of mealtime, you should have a moderate snack of carbohydrate along with some protein or fat (such as crackers and cheese, or nuts) after you have stabilized your blood sugar. This will tide you over to the next meal and prevent another reaction.

If you take insulin or any of the medications that stimulate insulin secretion, like sulfonylureas (see Appendix 3), you run the risk of not waking up when a reaction occurs or of becoming unconscious because hypoglycemia is not treated in time. This is not common with sulfonylureas alone, but it can happen. The people close to you should know what to do if they find you unconscious. Have a glucagon kit available and teach them how to use it in emergencies (glucagon is a hormone that causes your liver to release glucose into your bloodstream to wake you up.) If there is no glucagon, teach them to give you jam, jelly, or frosting instead. They should place some in your mouth and try to get you to swallow it without choking. If nothing is available in jellied form, they should give you small sips of fruit juice or soda pop (not diet soda). Tell them that as you recover you might be angry or confused. That's part of the reaction. If you don't recover consciousness within five minutes, they should call the paramedics or get you to an emergency room.

Make sure they know the difference between the symptoms of very low blood sugar (insulin shock) and very high blood sugar (diabetic coma). If you are in a diabetic coma, the only treatment they can administer is to call a physician and get you to a hospital immediately. If a doctor is not available, they should take you to an emergency room. Most likely, you will not have been feeling well for the last half-day or more. Diabetic

Insulin Shock (Low Blood Sugar)	Diabetic Coma (DKA) (High Blood Sugar)
Sudden onset (minutes to hours)	Gradual onset (days)
Pale, moist, sweaty skin	Flushed, dry skin
Shallow breathing	Deep, labored breathing
Normal breath	Fruity smell on breath
Rapid pulse	Usually rapid pulse
Low blood sugar	Very high blood sugar

coma is gradual in onset, and usually you feel ill, thirsty, and have to urinate frequently as the condition progresses.

Tell them to give you some carbohydrate to revive you if they're not sure whether you have low or high blood sugar. Low blood sugar can cause harm more quickly than high blood sugar.

Prevention

The best way to avoid low blood sugar is to maintain an awareness of your diabetes. Don't obsess about it, but acknowledge that it is a companion who refuses to be left behind. People who frequently suffer from hypoglycemia are often the ones who pretend they do not have diabetes. This lack of management doesn't work, and they often end up with vivid reminders of their condition.

You are more likely to have low blood sugar in certain situations. If you have been more active, delayed a meal, or eaten lightly, hypoglycemia will occur if you don't compensate for the change in routine. If these situations heighten your awareness, you will find that you automatically take the appropriate action. The light meal or the delay becomes a signal to eat a snack (unless blood sugar tests are high).

To adjust to an increase in activity level, take less insulin or increase your food intake. Through trial and error you will find the amount that's right for the kind of activities you are involved in. You will be able to hike or work in the garden all afternoon and maintain balance, avoiding both reactions and high blood sugar. Note that vigorous activities such as digging with a shovel, playing tennis, or hiking uphill can use nearly an entire meal's worth of calories in one hour.

Take another look at your meal plan if you're experiencing frequent hypoglycemia. If you eat slower-burning foods, you will have a more continuous supply of glucose entering the bloodstream. This is one reason that nutritionists recommend meals high in fiber and slowly absorbed carbohydrate.

Protein and fat burn even slower, but you still have to watch your total fat intake carefully.

As you become more aware of the physical sensations that precede hypoglycemia, you will be able to determine how much quickly absorbed carbohydrate you need to maintain normal blood sugar levels. You gain a sense of "dosage" with foods such as raisins, prunes, and fresh fruit. Sometimes you can just shift the order of your meal, eating fruit or other carbohydrate at the beginning of the meal rather than at the end. Anyone who has experienced a reaction that occurs while eating a meal that won't be absorbed for an hour knows the value of this practice.

Developing an Early Warning System

Sensitivity to the symptoms of hypoglycemia varies greatly among people. Some may be very aware of bodily states, noting the onset of hypoglycemia at a very early stage. Others may be so absorbed in day-to-day activities that they recognize a reaction only when sweat is pouring down their brows and their speech is slurred. You can take steps to increase your awareness and thereby your chances for survival.

One way is to make routine physical activities like brushing your teeth, shaving, or showering occasions for feeling your body rather than thinking about other things. Become aware of the sensation of temperature in various body parts, muscle tensions, the texture of whatever surface is in contact with your skin, or the feeling of your breath or pulse. (When you are still you can sense the pulsing of your whole circulatory system.) A good time for observing is when you are waiting for something to happen. Your body is always happening—no waiting necessary!

A more direct way of heightening physical awareness is to focus on everything you experience as you become hypoglycemic (and, of course, as you eat something). See how many different sensations you can notice, and make mental notes; the sensations may differ from time to time. This is also a good time to identify the more subtle changes that may be present during hypoglycemia unawareness.

Along with increasing body awareness, you can use blood testing to help determine when a reaction is near. When you note a physical change that might be signaling the approach of low blood sugar, check to see what your level actually is. If you are in the normal range (70–120 mg/dl), wait a few minutes and see if more distinct symptoms develop. (If you're at the lower end of the normal range, you're more likely to have a reaction.)

After you treat your reaction, try to remember how you felt leading up to it. If you write down the symptoms you had, next time you can bring your blood sugar levels up before stronger symptoms develop. And you can better avoid the possible rebound to high blood sugar levels if you overtreat.

Let Others Know

Don't be shy about letting people around you know you have diabetes. Your family, friends, and workmates need to know what your signs of low blood sugar are. Don't risk a situation dangerous for you—and difficult for others—because you feel embarrassed. It's going to be a lot more embarrassing—and potentially life threatening—if no one knows what is going on. Someone else may notice the signs of your hypoglycemia long before you do. If someone close to you thinks you are having a reaction, make it easy for them to help you.

Make sure you get what you need. Don't worry about inconveniencing others. You are not expressing a simple preference when you say, "I need to eat *now*." It can be hard to tell your friend who has made special plans, "I can't wait until we get to the beach to eat. Can we stop now? I'm having a reaction." But if you don't take care of yourself, your friend will have to. Most people will understand.

If you have to give a speech or make a presentation, test your blood sugar beforehand and eat a snack if you need to.

If you can't test, go ahead and have a snack anyway. The risk of temporarily higher blood sugar levels is certainly less than the risk of having a reaction at an important moment (especially if your performance involves physical activity.)

And always wear a diabetes I.D. bracelet or necklace and carry a card with details of your medication and insulin dosage. This could save your life.

Watch Out for the Hidden Gain

If you find yourself reluctant to treat early symptoms of low blood sugar, there may be some hidden gain for you in the reaction. For example, you may use it as an excuse to binge on desserts ("Oh, boy, a sweet treat! This is a pretty strong reaction. I must need a hot fudge sundae or apple pie à la mode").

The solution is simple: don't use a reaction as an excuse to do something you can already do. In this case, you're already allowed sweet treats—you just need to account for them in your meal plan. You'll feel much better if you don't have to go through a reaction to get some dessert!

Some of us use hypoglycemia as an excuse to express hostility we normally keep inside. Some of the nicest people rant and rage when their blood sugar levels fall too low. Anyone who suggests that they may need a few chocolate chip cookies becomes a target for their abuse. When it is all over, they blame their behavior on their diabetes. If this is your approach, learn to express your anger directly and appropriately instead.

Some people want others to take the responsibility for their low blood sugar. Not waking up from a nighttime reaction practically guarantees that someone else has to take care of you. This can become a way of testing a mate or a parent: "If you really love me, you'll save my life." It can also be a form of revenge, given the amount of stress the rescuer feels as he or she revives you. Ironically, the person who fails to take care of himself at night may be the very one who fights off all assistance during the day, insisting, "Don't you think I can take care of myself?"

Fred's Story

Fred, a man in my support group, experienced repeated nighttime hypoglycemia that had to be treated by his wife or the paramedics. He insisted he couldn't do anything about it and his wife was growing increasingly frustrated and angry. When he had a reaction during the day, he insisted on his independence and ability to take care of himself. But he never wanted to pay attention to the symptoms his wife would point out in the evening, often waiting until he was hypoglycemic before he would eat. It took the feedback of the support group to help Fred see what he was doing to his health and his marriage.

—Mary, 46

This is a delicate issue to work with. We want to be independent, yet we depend on food, medications, regularity of meals, family and friends, and doctors to help us handle our condition and its complications. And worst of all, in a very fundamental way, we cannot depend on our own bodies as others do. No wonder we declare our independence and act very dependent at the same time. Talk with your support group or counselor about ways to resolve your conflict.

Low Blood Sugar and Sex

One of the frustrations in the life of a person with diabetes occurs when the passion drains away just before or while making love, and low blood sugar takes the place of an orgasm. Your body makes the wise choice of preservation over reproduction and pleasure, but sometimes that's not easy to explain to your partner. This is another time when a pre-event blood test and extra food may be in order, especially if you tend to be an athletic lover.

CHAPTER 11

Handling Complications

"Complications?! I don't want to hear about them. That's too depressing."

If this is how you feel when you turn to this section, we can sympathize. After living with diabetes for over forty-five years each, we have experienced all the fears and uncertainties you might feel. However, we now know that complications are not an inevitable result of diabetes. How we live with diabetes can slow, prevent, and even reverse the development of its side effects. So learn how to prevent or minimize complications—today, tomorrow, next week, or whenever you're ready, but do it soon!

I want to know the risks I'm facing as a diabetic. Why stick my head in the sand and pretend I'm not worried? I tried that and it didn't work worth a damn. I kept hearing horror stories, anyway. I finally pushed through my fears and read about all the things that could happen to me. Glad I did. I found out what I could do to improve my odds for avoiding them.

—Marybeth, 50
40 years with diabetes, experiencing only minor complications

Neutralizing the Threat

Living with diabetes means living with the risks, and sometimes the reality, of complications. But you can delay or prevent them by learning about:

- changes in program and lifestyle that will reduce your risk.
- early warning signs that enable you to seek treatment if a complication begins to develop—both laboratory test results and symptoms you can recognize yourself (see Appendix 2, pages 234–235).
- treatments now available and under research for each complication.
- ways of reducing anxiety over the possibility of developing diabetic complications, or dealing with feelings that come up if they do begin.

Diabetes teaches us some challenging lessons. Perhaps the most challenging is how to live peacefully with physical and emotional risk. Can you accept that you're vulnerable and still live a full life? Can you face aging and mortality? Can you feel inwardly healthy, regardless of the state of your body? When you deal with the questions raised by complications, you grow as a human being.

If you're starting to feel anxious about the possibility of complications, find some relief in the following concepts.

1. Complications are not inevitable. There are ways to avoid the major complications of diabetes. When you read statistical reports on diabetic complications, you may believe you cannot avoid them. "Blindness is 25 times more common in individuals with type 1 diabetes" is a typical statement. Those are dramatic odds, but actually, fewer than one percent of us will lose our vision. The majority of people with diabetes do not become blind. Even without taking special precautions, you have a good chance of avoiding a major handicap.

Statistics are misleading—if not terrifying—for a very fundamental reason: they are based on an earlier era of diabetes care when the medical knowledge and tools we now have were not available. It was also a time when individuals were much less interested in a healthy lifestyle. But recent results have shown that the statistics for the present generation of those with diabetes can be improved.

2. You can reduce your level of risk by improving your diabetes self-care program.

- Maintain better control of blood sugar and blood pressure.
- Eat healthfully and lose weight if necessary.
- Live an active lifestyle.
- Practice stress management.
- If you smoke, quit.
- Get the amount of sleep and rest you need.
- Take a daily multivitamin.

You can increase your odds by the way you live. The risk is still there, but it is much smaller.

3. Treatment for most complications is becoming more effective. In many cases, complications can be reversed or reduced, especially when detected early. If a complication develops, you are more likely to find a treatment that will reverse or limit its advance. This is especially true if you are aware of its symptoms and seek treatment early. Thousands of people with diabetes avoid disability thanks to laser treatment, kidney transplantation, early treatment of foot disorders, aggressive management of high blood pressure and heart disease, and other new developments.

The main point about complications is that there are no guarantees. You aren't automatically going to experience them, and you aren't necessarily going to be able to avoid them. Other factors that cause you to develop complications—your genetics, for example—are not under your control. However, by taking care of yourself now, you can greatly reduce your risk. (For a very simple overview of complications, including causes, prevention, early warning signs, and treatment, see Appendix 2, pages 234–235.)

Learn to do your best, and live well with uncertainty. Learn to cope with anxiety and maintain hope, no matter what happens. This challenge is not altogether different from the one the world at large makes upon us all.

Complications and Me

This exercise will help you learn how you really feel about the possibility of developing diabetic complications. Answer spontaneously, even though the feeling or belief that comes may seem "wrong."

1. What did you feel as you read the title of this chapter?

____

____

2. Which of the following statements describe(s) the way you have dealt with complications in the past?

☐ I don't want to think about the possibility of complications.
☐ I worry about them quite a lot.
☐ It makes me angry that diabetes could do that to me.
☐ I do everything I can to reduce the risk.
☐ I can do more to reduce the risk.

- ☐ I just do everything I want to, since I don't know how long I'll last.
- ☐ I probably spend too much time taking care of my diabetes.
- ☐ I feel depressed quite a bit.
- ☐ I feel guilty because I have not taken good care of myself.

3. I believe I will probably live to the age of ______

4. The complication I fear the most is

____

5. I believe:

- ☐ I will escape major complications.
- ☐ I am very encouraged by recent findings showing complications can be prevented.
- ☐ I will certainly develop a major complication.
- ☐ There is nothing I can do to change what will happen.
- ☐ If one complication develops, others will follow.
- ☐ If I become (or am) disabled in any way, my life will be damaged beyond repair.
- ☐ I will be able to learn to live well with the disability.
- ☐ I will be a burden to others.

I also think that complications:

____

____

____

My positive beliefs that neutralize any negative beliefs are:

____

____

____

6. Is there anyone close to you who keeps reminding you of what can go wrong? Who uses threats to motivate you? Have any of your doctors done this?

____

7. My present level of blood sugar control is __________. My level of care is _______ (See your questionnaire results on page 52.)

8. I intend to make the following improvements in self-care in the next months:

____

____

9. I can get support for my feelings about complications and for making changes from:

____

____

10. I do not intend to make any changes in self-care at this time because:

- ☐ I am already doing everything possible.
- ☐ I do not believe it will do any good.
- ☐ I do not feel I have the time and energy needed.
- ☐ I feel the changes would reduce my freedom or pleasure.
- ☐ I feel overwhelmed by the demands of diabetes.
- ☐ Other____

11. If someone you loved gave the reason(s) checked above for not improving their diabetes self-care, what would you say to that person?

____

Make an appointment with yourself to re-ask question 11 in a few months. Mark it on your calendar.

Reflect on your answers to these questions. Look for places you can change your beliefs or behaviors that will help you lessen the threat of complications. For example, if you do not have the time needed to improve your self-care program, ask yourself what changes in your life would give you that time.

Reducing Your Risk

A successful diabetes management program makes complications less likely and handles your day-to-day need for blood sugar control. Other ways you can reduce your risk are:

- Improve your blood sugar control, and continue improving it to the highest level you are comfortable with (ideally, an A1C less than 7%).
- Learn to handle stress well.
- Follow a healthy meal plan that is low in fat and high in fiber. Limit sweets and rapidly absorbed carbohydrates.
- Get moving! Engage in regular physical activity.
- If you are overweight, lose weight.
- Act to prevent high blood pressure by controlling stress and weight. Seek treatment for hypertension if your blood pressure is high (above 130/80).
- If you smoke, quit.
- Get the amount of sleep and rest you need.
- Know the warning signs for each complication.
- Take a multivitamin with antioxidants.
- Ask your doctor about taking low-dose aspirin to help prevent heart complications.

Except for the first item, this is virtually the same prescription for good health that doctors give those without diabetes. This prescription is especially important for you because each item will improve your odds of avoiding diabetic complications (or of limiting them if they have already started).

You may have already adopted some of the measures and need to make only a few changes. Or you may need to alter your life in every area. Begin where you feel most willing to change. If your sense of urgency is great, begin with blood sugar or blood pressure control, fundamental ways of reducing risk. Give yourself the best chance for a long and healthful life by following every risk-reduction step as well as you can.

Dealing with Anxiety

The best way to deal with anxiety about diabetic complications is to reduce your risk of developing them. But even if you are doing everything you can to reduce risk, or are in the process of learning to, you can still experience anxiety.

A useful skill to develop is the art of living well with uncertainty. For all the talk of risks and odds and possibilities, you simply cannot know whether you will end up with one or more diabetic complications. You can do your best to avoid them, but a degree of uncertainty is inevitable. Face the possibility that you will become disabled as a consequence of diabetes, but also realize the possibility that you will remain free of major complications. Decide to live well with yourself, no matter which path becomes yours, and return to the task of living well right now.

As you learn about complications, use stress-reduction techniques such as relaxation, meditation, prayer, and whatever else is effective for you. Learn the information in small doses, and give yourself breaks to focus on fun, positive aspects of your life. Participate in a diabetes support group or have conversations with others who have diabetes to help you deal with the feelings that come up. Find a good counselor if your feelings become overwhelming.

One reason for doing the questionnaire on page 164 is to help you explore your beliefs and attitudes about complications. Neutralizing negative beliefs and adopting a positive attitude can help relieve the anxiety, depression, or anger you may experience. For instance, a typical belief is, "I've been so out of control that I can't possibly avoid complications." This is a belief, not a fact. A more helpful belief is, "If I improve control now, I may still escape major complications."

If You Decide Not to Act Now to Reduce the Risks of Complications

You may feel unwilling at this time to make the changes in your life that will lessen the risk of complications. If so, it is important that you make this a conscious decision. Look at why you want to maintain your present level of self-care. Discuss them with someone you trust and explore them within yourself through writing, inner dialogue, prayer, meditation, or whatever method works for you.

Find a point of view that allows you to begin making the necessary changes, while dealing with your reasons for not changing. For example, if lack of time is your reason for not changing, find ways to change that do not require additional time, or learn to use your time more effectively.

If you decide not to change, accept your decision and any anxiety that goes with it. You will also have to accept greater risk. Make a date with yourself in a few months to ask yourself again what you are willing to do to stay well. Love yourself enough to want to be well.

If Complications Develop

Diabetic complications usually show early warning signs (see Appendix 2, pages 234–235). First signs often appear in lab tests, or you may notice the signs yourself. Your doctor may notice them during a routine exam. You may shrug off the news, or you may find it very disturbing. But this "bad news" can provide the motivation to improve your self-care regimen. Taking action will enable you to delay or halt the progress of the disorder, and perhaps even reverse it.

Coping with the Emotional Impact

The onset of a major diabetic complication can be a crisis, no matter how well you handle it. It reminds you of your vulnerability. You may feel angry and frustrated if your excellent self-care has not prevented complications. You may be in denial, ignoring both the doctor's recommendations and your own feelings. You may withdraw while you absorb the impact of the news. You may feel doomed. You may throw self-care out the window and go on a food binge. At the same time such feelings arise, you might have to make serious decisions about treatment and lifestyle changes.

All of this creates a major challenge that demands your time, energy, and the support of others. You will live well through this crisis if you learn to deal with the many practical, emotional, and social demands it places on you.

Understand what your pattern of response to the diagnosis of a complication has been. If your response is negative, do not fault yourself for reacting this way. You've had to deal with a stressful piece of news. But recognize the limitations of this initial reaction and allow yourself to move on to a more functional response.

If a major body function is involved, such as loss of vision, amputation, or kidney failure, it is natural to go through a grieving process. You will find yourself going through a series of emotional reactions, rather than experiencing just one. Allow yourself to feel what you are feeling. If you are unable to function, ask for help.

Family and friends are often able to help. Immediate family members usually experience their own stress about what is happening to you, so it is best not to rely solely on them. (In some cases, their input may be so negative or fearful that it is better to seek support elsewhere.) Others who have dealt with complications will know what you are going through. They can help you sort things out at a practical level, and offer encouragement at the same time.

If informal support is not enough, you might want to see a psychologist or psychiatrist or a social worker who specializes in medical counseling. A diabetes educator who is trained in dealing with complications is also a good resource. (The American Association of Diabetes Educators provides a toll-free number for referrals, 1-800-TEAM-UP-4.)

The onset of a diabetic complication is a time when you gain a new appreciation of your internal resources for coping. Such a crisis often puts you in touch with your personal strength and spirituality. You may also gain encouragement from remembering those who helped you in the past. See page 186 for more techniques to help you handle your emotional responses.

Treatment and Self-Care

You will have to absorb new information, learn new skills, make important decisions, and change aspects of your life at this time. These changes may feel overwhelming, especially when you are dealing with your emotions. You can regain control of the situation if you define the tasks facing you. Break them down into manageable steps. Establish how much time is needed, what resources and support you will need, and what information you must acquire. By organizing the demands, you are better able to deal with them. (The questionnaire on page 173 will guide you through this process.)

You will probably be faced with decisions about treatment and regimen. In some cases, specialists will describe complicated procedures that can be difficult to follow. If you do not understand what is being recommended, ask for an explanation in language you do understand. If you still don't understand, ask your internist, family practitioner, or diabetes educator to help you. Ask if there are written materials or audiovisual aids describing the treatment. You need to understand what you are being asked to undergo.

You should know the risks of the recommended treatment. What are the odds for success? For a negative outcome? What will happen if you do nothing? Are there alternative treatments available? If you have any doubt about the treatment your doctor suggests, seek a second opinion from another physician with equivalent expertise. (Do not go to a general practitioner or an internist for a second opinion about eye treatment. You need an ophthalmologist, preferably one who specializes in retinal diseases or diabetic retinopathy.) If your doctor does not have much experience working with diabetes, you should probably find someone who does to guide the treatment of complications. Always ask your doctors how experienced they are in a treatment or procedure. For example, ask how many procedures were done in the last week or month.

In addition to prescribing a specific treatment, your doctor may suggest that you improve your self-care regimen at this time. Improvement in blood sugar control may help you handle the condition that has developed. It will also make other complications less likely to occur. You will need to proceed cautiously in tightening metabolic control if you have advanced retinopathy or kidney disease.

You will need to be cautious in your exercise and physical activity at this time, depending upon the specific complication you have. This is especially true if you are beginning an exercise program after a period of inactivity. Discuss exercise and physical activity with your doctor. You may want to enroll in a medically supervised exercise program that monitors your physical condition.

This is also a good time to improve your meal plan. Begin by eating more fresh vegetables and fruits, and cut down on animal and saturated fats. Monitor your carb intake to fit your meal plan. Add more beans, grains, and other high-fiber foods to your meals.

Diagnosis and Me

Take this questionnaire after you've been diagnosed with a complication. It will help you clarify what is happening, how you are responding, and what you need to do.

1. What diabetic complication(s) has your doctor diagnosed?

   ____

   ____

2. At what stage of development is the complication?

   ____

   ____

3. What treatment does your doctor recommend?

   ____

   ____

4. What risks are involved with this treatment?

   ____

   ____

5. What are the odds for a successful outcome?

   ____

   ____

6. What does your doctor think will happen if you do nothing?

   ____

   ____

7. What changes in regimen or lifestyle does your doctor suggest?

___

___

___

___

8. Do you think you will have trouble making these changes? (If so, see pages 27–30.)

___

9. Outline the steps needed to make these changes. Also include any decisions you need to make about treatment, or things you have to do to undergo treatment.

___

___

___

___

10. How are you coping with the diagnosis of the complication so far?

- ☐ I am trying to ignore what the doctor told me.
- ☐ I am ignoring my feelings.
- ☐ I am paying attention to my feelings.
- ☐ I am reading everything I can find about the complication.
- ☐ I am talking with people who have been through this.
- ☐ I am feeling withdrawn. I don't want to talk to anyone.
- ☐ I am worrying a lot and dwelling on the worst possible outcome.
- ☐ I am blaming myself and feeling guilty.
- ☐ I am living it up. I'll enjoy myself while I can.
- ☐ I am doing everything possible to take care of myself.

- ☐ I am becoming too dependent on my family and friends.
- ☐ I feel completely overwhelmed.
- ☐ Other________________________________

11. How would you like to change your reaction?

____

____

12. How are you feeling about the diagnosis?

- ☐ Angry
- ☐ Frightened or anxious
- ☐ Guilty
- ☐ Depressed
- ☐ Hopeless
- ☐ Hopeful
- ☐ Grief-stricken
- ☐ Calm
- ☐ Other________________________________

13. What support can you count on? (Name the people.)

- ☐ Family ________________________________
- ☐ Friends________________________________
- ☐ Diabetes network________________________
- ☐ Other support network ___________________
- ☐ Professional and religious counselors ___________
- ☐ Other________________________________

14. If you do not have enough support, what steps can you take to find the help you need?

____

____

____

____

CHAPTER 12

Managing Stress

When we are presented with physical or emotional challenges, we respond physically and emotionally with a set of responses called "the stress response." We need the stress response to function. It mobilizes us for action and organizes our defenses to maintain vital functions when we are ill or injured. But this can be a problem if you have diabetes. To protect your brain and ensure energy for action, your body will raise your blood sugar level when you feel stressed.

Sometimes I feel like I'm just going crazy. I have to work all day at a tough job, then come home and deal with the wife and kids, and somehow find time to check my blood sugar, exercise, and eat right. I feel like I'm going to explode.

—**Harry, 41**

Emotions can trigger the stress response as easily as a physical disorder. In fact, the body can't really tell the difference. An argument, a disappointment, or a thrilling discovery can cause a release of hormones that raise (or lower) your blood sugar. Frustration or depression that continues for days can cause elevated blood sugar levels throughout the period. If you overeat as a response to stress, your blood sugar levels can shoot even higher.

Poorly managed stress has a major impact on the health of everyone—not just the health of those with diabetes. Stress is believed to contribute to heart disease, high blood pressure, and cancer. Although other factors play a role in these conditions, reducing your stress level is likely to increase your ability to live well.

Stress and Diabetes

As people with diabetes, we have reasons to take special interest in the effects of stress.

- Simply having diabetes generates stress-inducing events.
- Physical and emotional stress can greatly affect our blood sugar levels.
- Chronic stress can contribute to the development of diabetic complications.

These three facts make an effective stress-management program a high priority for anyone with diabetes. If you follow such a program, you will be stabilizing your blood sugar levels by reducing the effects of stress on your metabolism. You will be lowering the risk of developing complications, and you will find it easier to live well with diabetes as you neutralize the stress of managing it.

Let's examine the three ways that stress affects diabetes.

1. Simply having diabetes generates stressful events.

How many simple events become stressful for us because we have diabetes? "Sorry, dinner's going to be a bit late." "I'm afraid your luggage got put on another plane." "Looks like that blister on your foot is infected." "No, there isn't a drugstore open here on Sunday." Our sense of security depends upon an amazing number of routines functioning smoothly. We are vulnerable to circumstances that may be trivial to others.

In almost every hour of the day, we must consider some aspect of our self-care, and we may be confronted with a significant diabetes-related problem. Even our sleeping hours may be disturbed by the shaking cold sweat of a low blood sugar reaction (an event of great physical stress).

These day-to-day stresses of diabetes can create strong feelings of anxiety because they remind us of something greater: the fear of diabetic complications. This is true whether we have type 1 or type 2 diabetes. No matter how much we may try to forget the possibility of blindness, kidney failure, or heart disease, our mind remembers that we are at risk. Anything that suggests this risk becomes a source of further stress.

Now is an excellent time to practice stress management. Check to see how you responded to what you just read. What changes can you detect in your body? Do you feel edgy, tense, nervous, or suddenly tired? How is your mind responding? Do you want to stop reading to deny that you are at risk?

Close your eyes and say to yourself, "I am learning to take better care of myself. I am reducing the risks." Let the words relax you as you repeat them several times. If any other words try to deny what you are affirming, just hear them as static on an untuned radio station. This illustrates one way of reducing stress: replacing the thoughts that trigger it with more reassuring thoughts.

2. Physical and emotional stress can greatly affect our blood sugar levels.

Diabetes gives us added sources of stress, and we are more vulnerable to its effects. Physiologically, the stress response creates a powerful shift in hormone levels. It can raise, and sometimes lower, blood sugar levels to two or three times their normal level. A botched and painful drawing of blood by an incompetent lab technician can result in an artificially high test result because of the emotional stress you feel. Similarly, a scare while driving or a put-down from the boss can send blood sugar levels soaring. Learning how to manage stress can help prevent these highs and lows.

Use blood glucose testing to do your own research on emotional stress in diabetes. When you have had a difficult day, an argument, a fright, or a disappointment, check your blood sugar level. See if it is significantly higher or lower than what you would expect on the basis of the day's activity and food. Some people find that a stressful experience can raise their blood sugar to 400 mg/dl or even higher. Also, note whether you have reactions from particular types of stress, such as when you have expressed your feelings strongly. Keep notes on your observations in a section of your diabetes log. After a while, you will understand how your system responds to emotional stress.

Physical stresses such as infections, wounds, or burns are likely to have a powerful effect on metabolism, raising both blood sugar and ketone levels. These high levels, if uncontrolled, slow down healing and can result in medical emergencies and hospitalization. Blood sugar testing and adjusting insulin dosage can be lifesavers when we suffer severe physical stress.

People with diabetes who experience high stress levels often find that their blood sugar levels decrease when they take time to relax. A holiday or vacation can actually cause more low blood sugar episodes. This is due not only to any increased exercise you do on vacation, but also because fewer stress hormones are at work.

3. Chronic stress can contribute to the development of diabetic complications.

High blood sugar levels are thought to be the primary cause of complications, but there is growing evidence that stress also plays an important role. Heart disease, for instance, is strongly associated with poorly managed stress in the general population. With diabetes, high levels of stress hormones may contribute to such conditions as retinopathy. Stress is also a factor in high blood pressure, which in turn contributes to the development of numerous complications. Clearly, effective stress management is an important component in any program to reduce the risk of complications.

Understanding the Stress Response

Stress is an inherent part of living. When changes occur in our environment, our bodies react. There are similarities to these reactions no matter what the external stimulus (called the stressor) may be: a threat of physical attack, an emotional blow, a joyous event, a burst of energetic activity, or an actual injury or illness. The stress response is our body's attempt to maintain or restore healthful conditions to itself. Hormones are released, blood sugar levels rise, insulin becomes less effective, and you are ready for "fight or flight." Your energy is mobilized for an all-out effort.

This mobilization has a negative effect on blood sugar control, unless it is in preparation for a major physical event. Your pancreas is unable to produce enough insulin to remove the extra blood sugar stimulated by the stress. If this occurs, your next blood sugar check will be high. If you didn't know you were under stress, you might shake your head in puzzlement, saying, "But I didn't eat any more than usual!"

The effects of stress do not stop with those directly related to diabetes. Your muscles become tense. When you are unable to relieve this tension, headaches, back pain, and other muscular disorders can occur. Your digestive system becomes involved, with changes in the secretion of stomach acids, digestive hormones, and the muscle tone of the alimentary canal. Blood fat and cholesterol levels increase to provide energy for action. Pulse and blood pressure increase. The whole body participates in the stress response. If you don't take the steps to manage stress, the tension, hormones, glucose, fats, and other stress products stay at unnaturally high levels. Your health will suffer.

We don't even know if stress will raise or lower blood sugar levels in any particular person. But armed with your blood glucose test kit, urine ketone test strips, and logs, you can do the research that is most important: determine how stress affects you as an individual.

Note distressing or exciting events and periods; study your test results in relation to these events. See if there is a difference in blood sugar levels during a week when you are depressed and a week when you are happier than usual. What happens after a quarrel or a frightening episode? The following questions can help you determine how stress affects your diabetes.

1. Does stress seem to have much effect on your blood sugar levels? If so, do your blood sugar levels increase or decrease?
2. Does the type of emotion aroused influence the direction or amount of change in blood sugar?
3. What difference do you see between short, intense moments of distress and long, drawn-out episodes? What impact do you find from stress that extends for days or weeks at a time?
4. Are the effects on blood sugar levels different when you express feelings rather than hold them in?
5. Do you have positive tests for ketones in your urine after stressful incidents? If so, when?
6. How do attempts to cope with stress through self-gratification (such as overeating, drinking, and not exercising) disrupt control?
7. What overall patterns do you see in the ways you respond to stress?

As you understand more about how stress affects your control of diabetes, you will be better equipped to handle it. You will know that you need to check your blood sugar level after certain experiences to see whether you need extra insulin. You will know whether you need to modify your insulin dose during times of increased or decreased stress. And you will know which stressful experiences you need to manage more effectively.

Recognizing Signs and Symptoms

Some of us are more aware of feelings and physical sensations and have no difficulty recognizing the signs of stress. But if you have trouble knowing when you are feeling stressed, you need to become more aware. Ignoring the effects of stress does not decrease its impact. And if you know when stress is building, you are better able to deal with it.

Acute Signs and Symptoms of Stress

- Pounding heart, rapid pulse
- Trembling, shaky
- Dry throat and mouth
- Difficulty concentrating
- Change in blood sugar level
- Emotional and physical tension
- Sweating
- Easily startled
- Diarrhea or frequent urination
- Indigestion
- Compulsive eating
- Tension headache

At times, you may mistake a low blood sugar reaction for a stress response, or vice versa, because the symptoms overlap. You may have signs of low blood sugar such as blurred or double vision, tingling or metallic taste on the tongue, and confused thinking. If in doubt (and if you cannot test your blood at the time), eat some carbohydrate and see if your symptoms decrease.

Chronic Signs and Symptoms of Stress

General irritability
Easily fatigued
Depression
Loss of appetite
Anxiety
More accidents and mistakes than usual
Nervousness
Migraines
Nightmares
Missed menstrual periods
Stuttering
Chronic muscular pains
Insomnia

Relax and Recover

There are three main ways to manage stress.

A. Reduce the frequency of stressful incidents.

1. Make changes in your family, social, or work situation. You may find it easy to act on your environment, requesting changes in the people and conditions that produce stress for you. For the less assertive, you may be able to withdraw from whatever it is that distresses you. For instance, you might have a doctor who doesn't listen to you or who tries to motivate you with fear. Explain how that approach affects you, and ask for changes. If your physician doesn't respond, or if you choose to avoid the confrontation, change doctors.

2. Change beliefs and emotional patterns that trigger stress for you. Focus on yourself, using the source of stress to determine the areas of your personality that need change. With the same insensitive doctor, you might discover that the cause of your stress is the belief "No one thinks anything I say is important." By eliminating this belief, you will reduce your stress and find it easier to speak with more confidence. Similarly, you can work with feelings of repressed anger triggered when an authority figure ignores you. By detaching yourself from such responses, you learn to use the energy they release.

3. **Learn skills that allow you to function more effectively.** Often the source of distress is a sense of inadequacy that can be corrected by performing tasks that are important to us. This might involve learning, working, relating, or simply enjoying life. For example, you might overcome your physician's resistance to listening by taking a workshop in assertiveness training or communication skills (assuming this is not the only relationship in which you have difficulty getting your point across).

4. **Prepare for events likely to be distressing.** We often do this negatively by imagining everything that can possibly go wrong, sometimes in great detail. This skill of visualization can be turned into a positive resource by relaxing and imagining what goes well at the potentially stressful event. Imagine yourself performing with strength and clarity. Go through the experience in detail several times, especially if you see yourself faltering. Visualize yourself performing successfully, but don't try to use the visualization as a map when you get to the actual event. Real life calls for spontaneous, not rehearsed, action.

B. Reduce the intensity of your stress response by learning to relax.

Your body knows how to relax, but sometimes your mind forgets to use this essential skill. When you practice it during a distressing incident, you can lessen the physical impact of the event. Even if you forget to relax until afterward, you still benefit from releasing the tension that developed under stress. A relaxed body deals with stress more effectively and provides the best conditions for creative problem solving. Some studies indicate that people with diabetes who regularly practice relaxation improve their metabolic control. It also just feels better to be relaxed! Try some of the relaxation techniques below.

1. **Breathing exercises.** Begin by observing your breathing. What part of your torso are you using? How deep or shallow is your breathing? How fast? Are you holding your breath unconsciously? Next, focus on the air moving through your nostrils. Follow the air into your lungs, feeling your chest and stomach expanding and contracting with each breath. Focus now on each exhalation, imagining that the air is carrying tension out of your body. If you are alone, sigh or hum gently with each breath. Finally, focus on each inhalation, imagining new energy coming into your body with the air.

2. **Visualization.** This involves all of your senses to produce relaxation. For example, imagine warm water flowing gently across your tense muscles. Imagine each breath carrying tension out of your body. Or imagine a fragrant garden filled with the sounds of birds singing. Another method is to let your mind return to a specific time when you felt happy and deeply relaxed. Relive the event in as much detail as you can. Your body releases tension in response to this visualization process.

3. **Autogenics.** This technique uses words to instruct the body to relax. By telling yourself that your arms and legs are becoming heavier, and then warmer, you are suggesting that the results of relaxation are beginning to take effect. As you repeat the phrases, your body responds by relaxing further. When our minds talk, our bodies listen. For example, repeat each phrase slowly (and silently) five or six times:

- "My right arm is becoming heavier."
- "My left arm is becoming heavier."
- "My right leg is becoming heavier."
- "My left leg is becoming heavier."
- "My right arm is becoming warmer," and so on through the other limbs.

4. Massage. This can relax tense muscles, as well as lead to a sense of well being. Self-massage of temples, neck, shoulders, feet and calves can relieve tightness and pain. Learning specific acupressure points increases the effectiveness of massage.

5. Acupuncture. This technique, while not something you would typically do to yourself, can be very relaxing. Many people go to an acupuncturist for regular "tune-ups" that are reported to last several weeks to months. Five-Element acupuncturists, who focus on the spirit, are perhaps most suited for these tune-ups, although all acupuncturists deal with stress.

6. Music. Quiet and peaceful music can be used to create a relaxing environment. (In fact, relaxing music might help you work with this book.) Our bodies respond to excess noise with tension, but they often relax when the sounds around us are tranquil.

7. Meditation and prayer. Meditation is a centuries-old means of contacting inner sources of strength and calmness. Look for a meditation class at your local Y or rec center. Among the numerous approaches to meditation, one of the easiest to learn is called mindfulness. With this, you step back from the constant flow of thoughts and sensations and simply watch the parade.

- Find a posture you can maintain comfortably for 10–20 minutes without moving. Balance your body so you are not leaning forward, backward, or to the side. (Or lie down if you can stay awake.)

- Begin with awareness of the breath passing through your nostrils, and focus on this sensation. Let each breath remind you to observe the flow of thoughts, feelings, perceptions, and body sensations. Just watch, without commenting on or judging what you see.
- The value of this is you forget to "just watch" and you become immersed in the process of thinking and feeling. You forget even the simple task of sensing each breath. Then your breathing reminds you to detach and step back again.
- You move between watching and marching along in the parade of your mind. Gradually, the periods of watching become longer and the mind grows quieter.

Prayer may be viewed as meditating through words, directing your awareness to a sense of unity and connectedness. Some people envision their words being received by a deity; others imagine them joining the wholeness of the universe.

C. Become more active physically.

Since the stress response prepares us for physical activity, exercise is an ideal way to harness the physical changes produced by stress. Try running up and down stairs after you learn you will not get that hoped-for promotion. Jog or dance after a quarrel with your lover. Thirty to 60 minutes of moderate to brisk physical activity will use the adrenaline and begin lowering blood sugar levels. (If you have very high blood sugar because of stress, you may need extra medication or insulin.)

CHAPTER 13

Getting Support

I always felt lonely and a little weird, like I was the only diabetic in the world who lied to her doctor or ate lemon meringue pie. The only thing worse than my guilt was my depression over feeling so out of control. I didn't think anyone could understand what I was up against, until I went—unwillingly—to a diabetes support group. For the first time I got to talk to people who were struggling with the same issues that had me down. They taught me I could do something to get myself under control.

—Jean, 59

Diabetes is a demanding companion that can isolate you from others. Your friends and relatives may have little understanding of the frustrations and challenges you face. You may feel that you would only bore them with the countless details of self-care you have to stay aware of every day. You need support from those who understand diabetes to help you cope with your feelings, answer your questions, and help you take the best possible care of yourself.

Support from other people with diabetes is especially important when you decide to improve your level of management. The experiences, knowledge, and understanding of others who have gone through this process make the path much easier. They can help you see when you are trying to move too fast or when you are forgetting something important. They can also offer encouragement and practical tips. This type of help is an excellent complement to your medical team's support.

Those who are close to us need support as well. Being the partner or parent of someone with diabetes has its own unique demands. Finding a loved one unconscious or watching someone consistently overeating can be incredibly stressful. Support groups can really help spouses and parents learn, relax, and feel encouraged.

Creating a Support Network

There are informal and formal ways to set up a support network. Here's how to begin informally networking.

1. Start asking around to find people who function as diabetes networkers. Networkers are special people who love the process of making connections. They are often storehouses of information on people, resources, and meetings. "You're trying to get control of your eating? Talk to Joe Dodds. He's winning that battle and can really help you." "You're afraid of laser treatment and keep putting it off? Joan Mason can tell you how she overcame her fear." Don't feel that it is an imposition to ask for help. Most people enjoy an opportunity to help someone, especially when they share a common interest in diabetes.
2. Talk to your friends, relatives, doctors, diabetes educators, pharmacists, and clinics or hospitals with diabetes education programs. Tell them you want to contact people with diabetes who have positive attitudes and can encourage you. You may have to make a number of calls before you

start getting positive responses. Some doctors are appropriately protective of their patients, and some people with diabetes avoid others completely. Be prepared to persevere!

3. Contact your local American Diabetes Association chapter and ask if they sponsor any educational or support programs for people with diabetes. Also ask if there is anything else available in your area (or call the ADA information line, 1-800-DIABETES). Even general educational meetings are good places to meet other people with diabetes and begin building your diabetes network.

Soon you will have several people you can call when you need support or information. Perhaps occasional telephone contact or conversation over a diet soda or cup of coffee will satisfy your need for support. You'll go through a sorting process, dropping out of contact with complainers and forming friendships with others. You will soon be giving support to others, sharing news about diabetes care, a friendly drugstore, or an effective doctor. When you encourage another, you encourage yourself.

Often, you will be able to offer guidance or information well suited to someone else's needs. However, there will be times when there is little you can do. Don't feel that you must always have an answer. Your responsibility is to listen, show that you care, and share what you know. Sometimes "You'd better talk to your doctor or diabetes educator about that" is the most useful thing you can tell someone. As your network grows, you will be able to suggest others who can help with particular problems.

Developing a Support Group

Informal networking can provide very effective support, especially for people who are uncomfortable in groups. A formal group, however, offers certain bonuses. You can obtain feedback from a variety of points of view, and you have a larger body of experience to draw upon. A group can bring in guest speakers or even set up a training program dealing with aspects of diabetes management. Also, a group is usually more effective than individuals in handling a crisis such as the development of complications.

A support group is most effective when it is part of an ongoing network. If members feel free to contact one another between meetings, support is always available. Members maintain contact even when they are not able to attend every meeting. The meetings themselves are more relaxed, since they are only one of several times of sharing.

If you find no existing diabetes support group to join, you can start one by following the networking steps just described. Ask the people you contact if they are interested in creating a group. Find out what they are willing to do, what they want out of the meetings, and how often they would like to meet. You'll find some people who enjoy organizing and leading meetings, and others with practical skills such as typing or access to e-mail or copying machines. Share the work load so that you do not have to carry the entire burden. Be clear about the tasks people are assigned and specify when they need to be completed. "You're willing to call or e-mail Sarah, Phil, Joan, and Larry? The meeting is on the tenth, so can you do that by the second?"

You may want to proceed informally, or you may prefer to set up a coordinating committee from the beginning. Two or three other members are enough to work with you to organize the group, plan meetings, and develop other activities. It will become clear which decisions need to be made by the whole group and which by the committee. Some groups want to share the organizational tasks and decisions, and others prefer to use most of their meeting time for support and learning. In your initial conversations with potential members, you will get a sense of how they feel about this question. It can be explored at length in the first meeting.

Structuring Leadership

Establish a positive tone at the first meeting (this helps ensure that there will be a second meeting!). The details of this first meeting depend upon the wants and needs of the group. First, ask how the members want the group to be led.

- **Shared leadership.** The group will work together to develop guidelines, structure, and topics. The strength of this approach is that it encourages a high level of participation and responsibility. It reflects the level of individual responsibility demanded by diabetes. However, if some group members are dealing with major problems, they could find it difficult to assume this role.
- **Committee leadership.** A coordinating committee is responsible for defining initial guidelines and structure of leadership. This method is appropriate if you sense those coming to the first meeting are shy. The discussion leader briefly describes the proposed structure and asks for approval or recommendations for change. It is then possible to begin the support work. With good topics for initiating discussion, group members can quickly experience the value of being in a support group. However, it may take more effort to involve them in keeping the group going.
- **Outside leadership.** If you or the other members lack confidence in a self-directed group, a counselor or social worker might be hired to lead the first few meetings. Look for someone experienced at facilitating groups and willing to build the group's capacity to function on its own. A local college, hospital, or public health department can help you find such a person, who might even be willing to volunteer their time. If not, the group will have to be willing to collectively pay the leader.

After choosing a leadership structure, everyone in the group should answer the following questions.

- What do you want out of the group?
- What do you want to avoid?
- What guidelines for discussion are important to you?
- What are you willing to do to help the group function?

Support Group Guidelines

After a thoughtful discussion, you may find it helpful to propose the following guidelines. Your group will want to adopt some or all of these. Type them up and read them before each meeting. Clearly stated guidelines help instruct new members and remind old members of the group's basic values and meeting format.

1. We are here to support one another in facing the challenge of living well with diabetes. By helping one another, we help ourselves. We intend to maintain a positive climate for discussing our experiences, feelings, problems, and solutions.
2. We will feel free to share any information about ourselves within the group, but we will not disclose anything we hear to people outside the group.
3. We will respect one another's right to remain silent as much as his or her right to speak. And we will be sure to create opportunities for the silent to speak.
4. The proper care of diabetes differs from person to person. We will remember that programs are individualized and not try to advise someone else on the basis of our own choices.
5. If we hear something that suggests possible changes in our own regimen of physical care, we agree to discuss such changes with our physician before acting.

6. If we feel anyone is passing on misinformation, we will not be afraid to challenge the information. When there is a difference of opinion or doubt, we will determine the facts with a health professional.
7. One of our functions is to share feelings. When we do this, we will give support but avoid interpretation and analysis. If any of us experiences deep emotions during the meeting, we will allow room for this. At the end of the meeting, one of us will check with the person to be sure they are okay.
8. We will feel free to express anger, but not to direct it at other group members.
9. Many of the topics we discuss at an informational level may arouse strong feelings and stress reactions. When any of us senses stress or tension, we will feel free to ask for a moment of silence to calm our emotions. When the group stress level is high, we will take time for guided relaxation or another stress-reduction technique.
10. When one person is discussing a problem, we will encourage that person to find his or her own answers before offering ours. When we make suggestions, we will do it gently, without pushing.
11. If any of us is an alcoholic or drug user, we agree to come to meetings only when we are sober or straight.
12. If any of us decides to stop coming because we can't handle the issues the group discusses or the way the group functions, we will discuss our reasons in the meetings or contact someone in the group and give feedback on what is causing the difficulty.
13. Having diabetes challenges us to learn the lessons of life with which we are faced. We are together to support this learning.

These guidelines imply that all members can share many of the leadership functions in a group. If each person takes responsibility for maintaining discussion, awareness of stress levels, respect for feelings, and other questions of process, the meetings will practically run themselves. When there is an understanding of the group's guidelines, it is possible to function without a discussion leader.

It can also be effective to designate one person discussion leader, or facilitator, for each meeting, with the role rotating to another member each time the group meets. When a different member handles this job at each meeting, the whole group becomes experienced leaders.

Leading Effective Meetings

To lead an effective support group meeting, the facilitator can do the following things.

- **Encourage introductions.** At the beginning of the meeting, members introduce themselves by describing their relationship with diabetes and sharing something about their life outside diabetes. They can also mention subjects they would like to discuss during the meeting. The facilitator should list subjects on a chalkboard or large pad of paper. It is also helpful to know who has type 1 or type 2 diabetes and who is a parent or partner of a person with diabetes.
- **Start the discussion.** The facilitator can read the topic list and ask the group what it wants to discuss first. If the list is short, the facilitator can assign a subject, such as "the most useful thing I've learned about living with diabetes is . . ." or "how has diabetes improved my life?" It is surprising how willingly most people talk when such simple questions are presented.
- **Guide the discussion.** Sometimes meetings flow spontaneously, with little need for guidance from the facilitator. However, there are times when some direction is needed. One person may be cut off prematurely; a quiet "I'm not

sure Francis was finished speaking" will return the floor to the speaker. There may be shy members in the group who will say little or nothing during the meetings. The facilitator can open space for them by saying, "do any of those who have not said much want to speak?" Allow these members time to speak up, but do not pressure them. They may prefer to just listen for a while, and learn from other's experiences.

- **Set a positive tone.** A support group is more attractive if members emphasize abilities rather than disabilities, and solutions rather than problems. Members need room to describe the difficulties they experience, but they should be encouraged to overcome these difficulties rather than be victims to them. Ask questions in such a way that they elicit positive responses, such as "how do you deal with your feelings about diabetes?" rather than "what problems does diabetes cause?"
- **Stay aware of stress levels and strong feelings.** Many of the issues discussed at a support group can raise stress levels. The facilitator and group members watch for signs of stress, such as a tendency to quickly change the subject or give in to nervous laughter. It is always appropriate for a group member to ask, "is anyone else feeling anxious?" The group can do a "stress check" to see how members are reacting to the discussion. If enough group members are uncomfortable, the facilitator can lead a relaxation exercise (see pages 186–187). By doing this, members learn to be aware of and manage stress as it occurs. This also makes participation in the group a more positive experience.
- **Avoid misinformation.** Members must feel free to challenge information they believe to be inaccurate or incomplete. Keeping the facts straight is important. A self-led group may want to ask a doctor or diabetes educator to answer questions between meetings.

- **Handle difficult members.** If the facilitator lacks the necessary assertiveness to confront a member who dominates the discussion, drains the group with complaints and negativity, or sarcastically criticizes others, one thing to do is refer the difficulty to the group: "Jim seems to have a lot to say tonight. Does anyone else want to say anything?" Or suggest doing something that will change the tone: "Betty has pointed out a few things she doesn't like about doctors. I'd like to hear if any of you have anything good to say about your doctor." Or just say, "I'm frustrated. It sounds like everyone's doing everything wrong, according to Cliff."
- **Evaluate and close.** At the end of the meeting, each member describes what they most appreciated about the evening's discussion and mentions any changes that would improve the sessions. This feedback keeps the group on task.

Meeting Format

Support group meetings can follow a variety of formats. Each facilitates a different type of discussion, so it is good to vary the format occasionally. Some of the possibilities include the following ideas.

- **General discussion of questions and concerns.** Members can bring these up at the beginning of the meeting.
- **Sessions organized around a specific topic.** The coordinating committee can choose the topic in advance, or the group can decide the topic at the beginning of the meeting.
- **Discussion in subgroup.** Some subgroups are those on insulin and those on medication, family members with and without diabetes, or couples and singles.
- **Discussion in pairs.** The group can break up into pairs to discuss topics or just get better acquainted. This is important for people who are more comfortable talking one-on-

one than in groups. When the group reassembles, members can summarize their learning from the more intimate conversation.

- **Question-and-answer or instructional periods with a guest speaker.** A nurse practitioner or psychologist can give instruction in stress management for diabetes. You might ask a physician to answer questions such as "How can we most effectively use our office visits?" A dietitian might be asked to describe new research affecting nutrition and diabetes. (Guest speakers can be effective early in the development of a group to enlist new members.)
- **Watching films related to diabetes.** This is a great way to focus discussion. Ask hospitals, clinics, or your local ADA chapter how to obtain these.
- **Social events.** Have parties, picnics, and potlucks to share favorite recipes.

Topics for Discussion

Keep the following list on the back burner and turn to it if your group needs inspiration.

- ☐ How has diabetes been my teacher, helping me learn about living?
- ☐ What attitudes, beliefs, or skills have helped me cope with diabetes?
- ☐ What do I wish I had known about living with diabetes at the beginning?
- ☐ What benefits do I receive from diabetes?
- ☐ What are three things I like most about myself? How do they (or how could they) help me deal with diabetes?
- ☐ What attitudes and skills do I need to learn to deal with diabetes better? How can I learn them?
- ☐ How does diabetes affect my relationships, both intimate and casual?

- ☐ How did I feel when I first learned I had diabetes?
- ☐ What can I do to create a more effective relationship with my doctor and health care team?
- ☐ Given my need to respect the demands of diabetes, what can I do to improve the quality of my life?
- ☐ How can we cut the costs of managing diabetes?

When Support Groups Are Not Enough

Anyone with diabetes may encounter problems that require professional mental health assistance. Our support system may be weak, or the particular challenges we meet may require the aid of someone with professional training. Some of the signs of needing to see a professional (a counselor, social worker, psychologist or psychiatrist) include:

- Chronic depression.
- Repeated self-destructive behavior such as "forgetting" insulin, going on frequent eating binges, and not learning to handle insulin reactions.
- A sense of helplessness that blocks learning and action.
- Unwillingness to ask for help from an informal support system.
- Participation in negative family or social situations that detract from self-care.

If you feel you need more support than your network or group can give, don't hesitate to get it. Congratulate yourself on being willing to do whatever is necessary to achieve health, rather than thinking something else is wrong with you.

Working with Your Health Care Team

Of all chronic medical conditions, diabetes probably has the most sophisticated, well-developed team of health professionals dedicated to helping you learn about and manage the disease. You need to play an active role in choosing the members of this team and working with each one to help you stay well.

It is your responsibility to convey your needs, concerns, questions, and problems to individuals on the team. You need to speak up when you:

- do not understand something you are told.
- feel like too much is being said at once.
- think you will have difficulty carrying out a recommendation.
- do not agree with something you are told.
- want to know if there are alternatives to the recommended plan.

It is your health professional's responsibility to communicate the care options available to you. They should use words you understand, speak slowly enough for you to follow, and write down or provide printed information about their recommendations. They should outline the risks and benefits of alternative courses of action and explain any side effects of recommended tests, medications, procedures, or treatments. Then you need to ask questions, absorb the information, and work your self-care program.

Your team will consist of the members below.

- **Doctors.** Most likely, your primary care giver is either a family physician or an internist. Your doctor may have special interest or expertise in diabetes. There are also subspecialists—endocrinologists and diabetologists—who have special training in diabetes. Any of these doctors can help you live well with your diabetes. You have the right to choose a doctor you like, trust, and understand. You may want one who is more responsive to your individual needs, more knowledgeable about treatment options available, and more willing to work with you. These qualities can be more related to the doctor's personality than to training. Don't feel guilty if you decide to change doctors because you want a better relationship. If complications develop, your physician may refer you to a specialist in the area of your complication.

- **Ophthalmologists (eye doctors), podiatrists (foot doctors), and dentists.** Diabetes can affect you from head to toe. You need to see an ophthalmologist at least once a year for preventive purposes. You should be sure that your dentist and podiatrist are aware that you have diabetes. It will affect the signs and symptoms they look for and the kind of treatment they may give you. It is wise to have regular (yearly, and more often, if recommended) preventive maintenance on your teeth and gums and your feet.
- **Diabetes educators.** This category includes nurses, nurse educators, nurse practitioners, dietitians, nutritionists, patient educators, and exercise specialists. These specially-trained people can teach you what you need to know about living with diabetes. Look for people with CDE after their names. That stands for Certified Diabetes Educator and means the person had to pass a comprehensive exam. Some physicians are even CDEs.
- **Counselors, social workers, psychologists, and psychiatrists.** These professionals are available to help you with crises or difficult changes that you wish to make in your life. They can help you overcome resistance to following the diabetes care program you choose. They can also help you deal with crises, such as the onset of complications. To find someone who specializes in diabetes or other chronic illness counseling, contact your local chapter of the American Diabetes Association or call 1-800-TEAM-UP-4.

- **Pharmacists.** Pharmacists are extremely helpful in providing information on medications and how they affect diabetes. They can also inform you about insulin and the selection and use of a wide variety of diabetes products.

Your health care team will monitor your progress over time. Make sure you understand what tests you need and what the results were. You may find the following chart helpful. You can use this to track your own progress. Ask your team members if they are using a similar record.

Evaluations	Date of Visit
Review daily blood glucose records (every visit) My target (before meals): _____ (after meals): _____	_____ _____ _____ _____
Measure blood pressure (every visit) My target: _____	_____ _____ _____ _____
Weight (every visit) My target: _____	_____ _____ _____ _____
Foot exam (every diabetes care visit)	_____ _____ _____ _____
Dilated eye exam (every year)	_____ _____ _____ _____
A1C (every 3 months) My target: _____	_____ _____ _____ _____
Microalbuminuria (every year) My target: _____	_____ _____ _____ _____
Triglycerides (every year) My target: _____	_____ _____ _____ _____
HDL/LDL (every year) My target: _____	_____ _____ _____ _____
Flu shots (every year)	_____ _____ _____ _____
Pneumonia vaccine (on doctor's recommendation)	_____ _____ _____ _____

Support is available from the community of people who have and work with diabetes—those who best understand the meaning of living with diabetes. We can work together to deal with feelings, share information, and learn the skills needed for living well. This can happen through personal networking, support groups, or regular meetings with your health care team. You can feel supported on your journey to wellness—just tap into what's available!

PART FOUR

Women and Children Living Well

CHAPTER 14

Women and Diabetes

> When I told my mother I had diabetes, she cried. She thought that meant I could never have children. I told her she would have plenty of grandchildren!
>
> —**Sue, 18**

As a woman who has lived with diabetes for over 40 years, I know that it carries with it some special challenges. I have seen my blood sugars swoop when a period is approaching. I saw my insulin requirements nearly quadruple during my pregnancy. As I nursed my baby, I faced the additional challenges of low blood sugar as my body burned extra calories.

Those are physical issues. But there's another side to life with diabetes. I was unwilling to miss out on the fun and fulfillment of life, so I learned to be creative. As a teenager, I found that cheerleading and marching band

---

This chapter is written by Catherine Feste, a nationally recognized health motivation specialist, president of her own wellness consulting business, and the author of the best-selling book *The Physician Within* and *365 Daily Meditations for People with Diabetes* (ADA, 2004).

worked out fine if I hid LifeSavers in my uniform. Girl Scout canoe trips were not a problem if I kept insulin, syringes, testing strips, and carbohydrates in airtight plastic containers that would float. These early successes gave me the confidence as an adult to ski in the Rocky Mountains.

Living well as a woman with diabetes requires adapting to certain physical requirements without sacrificing quality of life. It's a constant balancing act. This chapter discusses the major physical issues unique to women with diabetes. It also explores some emotional and spiritual concerns associated with the condition.

Physical Factors

Diabetes presents women with special challenges during pregnancy, menstruation, and menopause. The interactions between blood sugar and hormone levels during these times affect our blood glucose regulation. Control, in turn, has a profound effect on pregnancy. Awareness of these effects will help you to manage both your diabetes and these aspects of your womanhood.

Menstruation

Although hormones definitely affect blood sugar levels, the effect is not the same in all women. Even more frustrating is the fact that the effect can vary in the same woman; some months your blood sugars may rise dramatically, and some months they may fall. Living well with this hormonal challenge requires a team effort. You need medical advisors on your team who are knowledgeable and experienced in diabetes as well as female issues. They will best understand the general effect of hormones on blood sugars.

Your job as a member of the team will be to record blood glucose levels accurately before, during, and after your menstrual periods. If you find a definite pattern, then together you can determine an appropriate course of action. If, for example, your blood sugar levels are consistently high the week before your period begins, then you may be able to successfully anticipate the increased need for insulin.

However, it may not be that easy if your needs cannot be anticipated. The hormonal impact may vary or your periods may be inconsistent. So you may choose to do nothing anticipatory, but deal with your fluctuating blood sugars in the same way you cope with any stress-related, unpredictable blood sugars. And be prepared! Carry what you need with you.

Birth Control

Since blood glucose should be under control before a woman becomes pregnant, it is important that a woman with diabetes practice birth control as soon as she becomes sexually active. Various methods are available. Choose one after considering its effect on your health as well as your personal preferences. Ask your diabetes doctor about using birth control pills.

Pregnancy

If you are pregnant, you need to make sure you are:

- seen and closely followed by a knowledgeable medical team experienced in diabetic pregnancies. Teams vary from center to center, but they usually include specialists in endocrinology, diabetology, obstetrics, dietetics, nursing, psychology, and social work or family counseling.
- educated about caring for diabetes and are motivated to act on what you learn.
- experiencing blood sugar levels within normal limits throughout the pregnancy. Research indicates that babies

in utero tolerate low blood sugars much better than they tolerate high blood sugars.

You should have a health assessment **before** you become pregnant. If you have existing complications, especially of the kidney and eye, learn about what effects the pregnancy might have on your health and the health of your baby. After an evaluation by a doctor extensively educated and experienced in both diabetes and pregnancy, you can make an informed choice about whether or not to attempt a pregnancy.

> When I decided to get married, my physician said to me: 'I think it's fine if you get married. But don't ever have children. Don't spread your genes around.' Because I am an educator, I believe that people ought to be given information and then make their own decisions. I felt that this doctor was giving me his personal opinion rather than information upon which to make a very important decision. So, my husband and I saw a genetic counselor who gave us not only information, but also a great deal of encouragement about the genetic issues involved. Appropriately informed about genetic issues and my good health, my husband and I chose to have a baby.
>
> **—Jill, 34**

Ask your doctor how many pregnancies in women with diabetes he or she has managed. Also ask how he or she manages them. If you need help finding a doctor, ask your local ADA chapter for a referral. Another essential element of a successful pregnancy is good health insurance. Even an uncomplicated pregnancy includes extra diabetes tests and visits to the medical team. A complicated pregnancy could include a lengthy hospitalization as well as intensive neonatal care for the baby. Make sure you have good health insurance before you become pregnant.

Throughout pregnancy, you should keep your blood sugars as nearly normal as possible. This helps you have a good outcome and keeps the baby's weight at a healthy level. Close control of blood sugars will mean that your lifestyle during pregnancy will be closely regulated. This may not be typical of your usual way of living. Most of us slide off our regimens occasionally, and some do so fairly frequently. Are you sure you're ready to do the work required to have a successful pregnancy? Actually, many women have reported that it turned out to be less of a challenge than they had anticipated. And your growing abdomen will serve as a constant reminder of why you're working so hard!

> Besides wonderful medical support, I was blessed with a supportive husband who gave me a steady diet of love and humor. As my abdomen increased, I began to wonder how much longer I should inject my insulin abdominally. Although my obstetrician gave me the answer "as long as it is both physically and psychologically comfortable," it was my husband's response that took the prize. He told me, "Just keep injecting in your abdomen until you hear someone say 'ouch'." Humor gives wonderful perspective.
>
> **—Cindy, 28**

Laboratory tests are an important part of your support in pregnancy. Each test and each visit to your medical team is an excellent reminder that you are not alone. Skilled people are doing everything they can to help you.

> I was extremely thankful to have an upbeat, 'human' medical team whose humor and warmth reinforced the excitement of a pregnancy instead of treating it like a high-risk, complicated medical problem. Whenever the seriousness of the situation did arise, I felt supported rather than fearful. For example, my diabetes doctor told me that any sign of infection, high sugars, or ketones should be reported immediately and not be left until tomorrow. It wasn't frightening to hear him say that, just reassuring to know that he would be there to help.
>
> **—Maureen, 24**

The baby's birth does not signify the end of the close working relationship between the mother and medical team. If you choose to nurse your baby, you must be well informed about your caloric needs for milk production as well as the ongoing balancing act with insulin. Throughout pregnancy, insulin requirements increase. Toward the end of a pregnancy, a woman may be taking two to three times as much insulin as in her prepregnancy days. At the time of birth, insulin requirements drop dramatically and a woman becomes extremely sensitive to insulin. Some women require no insulin immediately following delivery. The nursing mother may drop bedtime insulin entirely as her body burns many calories overnight for the production of milk. The teamwork continues. The baby is its newest member.

Because information on diabetic pregnancies is continually changing and growing, we encourage you to rely more on your medical advisors than on any printed information. Reflect on the issues. Make informed, responsible choices.

Vaginitis

Some women report that their diabetes was diagnosed when they went to see their doctor about severe vaginal itching. This problem is usually due to yeast infection. Women with diabetes have an increased incidence of yeast infections because yeast grows more rapidly in glucose found in urine. Your doctor can prescribe treatments for yeast infections, but prevention is better. Keep your blood sugars where they need to be. You might try adding yogurt with acidophilus to your meal plan—it decreases yeast infections in some women.

Menopause

At some point in middle age, women cease having periods. Because certain hormones are no longer present, the need for insulin usually drops. However, if the hormones are replaced, then insulin requirements will be affected by the estrogen. Higher doses of hormones require higher doses of insulin.

Day-to-day variations during menopause are far easier to handle with blood glucose monitoring. Some women experience profuse sweating during menopause and wonder if it is caused by hypoglycemia or by their "change." With blood testing, a woman can generally figure out what's happening and get in control of her life.

Emotional Challenges

As a woman with diabetes, you may have a distinct advantage over men with diabetes. You probably find it easier to connect with friends on an emotional level. To receive emotional support, you need to understand the language and be willing to engage in the process of both seeking and receiving it. The language of emotional support includes "I feel . . . I need . . . I am angry, fearful, or lonely because . . . It makes me feel so good when . . . ." Getting emotional support includes a willingness to begin conversations with phrases like these.

The process also requires time and an appropriate setting. A fifteen-minute commute on the way to work won't do it. An hour in a relaxed atmosphere like a restaurant or your home is more likely to allow the process to work.

If you don't want to talk to your friends about having diabetes, you might want to join a support group. Meeting others who have diabetes often creates an instantaneous bond that connects people on an emotional level. Check with your local ADA chapter or call 1-800-DIABETES for a local group. Take the step toward connecting on a feeling level. It may seem awkward at first, but keep at it. The rewards are great.

Dating and Marriage

Some women are reluctant to tell their dates that they have diabetes. If you are dating, consider the following scenarios.

1. Which situation would be better?
   a. You have an insulin reaction when you are with a date who knows you have diabetes.
   b. You have a reaction when you are with someone who hasn't a clue as to why your behavior is changed.
2. You are dating someone who needs to eat at a particular time. Would you prefer to have your date tell you that? Or, would you prefer to have him jeopardize his health to eat a fashionably late dinner?
3. Do you really believe that diabetes is such an awful disease that someone would not want to date you because of it?
   a. If your answer is yes, you should talk to a diabetes educator who can help you to adapt to diabetes and have a fun and full social life.
   b. If your answer is no, remember that you can influence the way your date thinks about diabetes. Present it positively, as a disease that can be controlled through a healthy lifestyle.

> A touching and reinforcing moment for me came at a party one evening when I overhead my husband say to a group of people: "The best thing that ever happened to me was marrying someone with diabetes. We live such a healthy life."
>
> **—Cathy, 54**

Most women fully expect to enjoy retirement with their spouses. They also expect to watch every hockey game of their children as they grow up. They look forward to graduation, weddings, and grandchildren. Without the challenge of a chronic condition, it is easier to deny that untimely death could ever rob them of their lifelong plans.

Besides a mighty important lesson about the uncertainty of life, diabetes can give one the gift of appreciating how precious life is. People blessed with the awareness that life is uncertain are in a unique position to enjoy life more fully. Time is more likely to be savored than wasted. All of life's experiences become a potential source of wonder.

> Just before I became engaged, I visited my doctor. Suddenly I had an urgent need to know the future. I wanted my doctor to look into a crystal ball and tell me what course my diabetes would take, so that I would have some idea of what "for better or worse" might mean to my husband. My doctor gently explained to me that no one knows what the future will bring. Perhaps the most profound lesson that diabetes has taught me is this: diabetes does not make life any more uncertain. It simply makes us more aware of the uncertainty of life.
>
> **—Claudia, 27**

Finding Your Balance

Although there surely are times when diabetes causes us to grapple with life's most profound issues, there are plenty of times when having diabetes is little more than a minor inconvenience. Balancing the emotions of those very different viewpoints is important to one's overall well being.

To follow a self-care regimen, we need to accept the seriousness of diabetes as well as our personal vulnerability. Then, we also need hope. We need to understand all of our options for health and act on them. Reflect on the issues that cause you emotional discomfort. Talk them over with a trusted advisor. Act to prevent problems, and promote health and well being. By taking positive action, you will gain an overall sense of control over your life.

Diabetes is ever present when I'm working too many hours and forgetting to balance my work with exercise (for the body). I have seen tests of 400 as a result of the distress of imbalance. It is tempting to curse my diabetes, saying "If it weren't for that darned diabetes, I could keep up the same pace as my friends do!" But then I look at the picture more carefully. What is really happening is this: diabetes tells me when life is out of balance and my body is asking me not to abuse it. Diabetes, in this case, is a blessing in disguise. In fact, I often find myself cautioning my friends who don't have diabetes to take better care of themselves. Although they know the harmful effects of stress, they don't have a tool (like my blood glucose meter) to tell them that their stress is harming them.

The heart of life is neither male or female, for it beats for all. The skills we need to live well with diabetes are the very same skills that anyone needs to meet the inevitable pain and challenges of life. To experience joy and soul-satisfying growth, we need to believe that diabetes has that gift to give. Great philosophers teach us that pain hollows us out, allowing us to hold more joy. They even suggest that pain holds as much wonder as joy. Indeed, joy and sorrow are inseparable in the same way that pain and growth often come together.

With maturity, we all become philosophers to some degree. If we can accept the philosophy that pain brings growth, then we have the foundation upon which to build a healthy life. Nietzsche said that people who have a *why* to life can bear almost any *how*. With this belief, we accept diabetes as one more building block of life.

Children and Diabetes

To live well with childhood diabetes calls for a unique partnership between you and your child, one that can enrich and deepen your relationship. You can learn together and grow together as you meet the demands of this condition. With a preteen, especially, you become a source of information and guidance as you learn about diabetes. At the same time, you respect and support your child's growing capacity for self-management and decision making.

> I liked it when I could do my own blood sugar testing. It made me feel like a grown-up.
> —**Caryn, 6**

Many of the techniques for living well described in this book apply to your life as well as your child's. Your maintenance of psychological health, good diet, and exercise programs becomes a model for your child. This is the very best way of teaching—to be what you want your child to become. With this understanding, taking care of yourself helps both you and your child. And you avoid the useless martyr role—sacrificing yourself for someone else's well being.

Use the tips for stress management and coping in Chapter 12, and find a support group for parents through your local chapter of the American Diabetes Association. Parents with experience can help you cope with your problems and guide you in handling the problems that come up with your child.

If your child has type 1 diabetes, you may feel a special urgency to learn how to help your child manage diabetes. But the current epidemic hitting children and teenagers is not type 1 diabetes, but type 2. There has been an alarming increase in the number of children diagnosed with type 2 diabetes in the past few years. What's behind this? Two things: poor eating habits and decreased physical activity. If your child is overweight and doesn't like to move around much, you and your child need to take action as soon as possible. Read Chapter 8 to find out how to help your child eat better, and start an easy, regular physical activity program like one in Chapter 9.

Living well with youthful diabetes demands a balance between the lives of all the family members and an adaptation to the unique pattern of the individual family. Different families have very different patterns concerning responsibility, decision making, participation, emotional support, health practices, and other areas important to diabetes care. You must find a way of dealing with the demands of diabetes that fits your family's patterns. But you may need to change patterns that unintentionally undermine your child's ability to live well. He or she may find it difficult to follow a healthful lifestyle if the rest of the family eats an unhealthy diet, doesn't exercise, and handles stress poorly. Becoming responsible for his or her own care will be hard if the parents are either too protective or too dominating.

Your Family Profile

To identify your family's patterns, explore your answers to this questionnaire. You can gain insight into your own family's patterns and how they may affect your child with diabetes.

1. How are decisions made in your family?

Do you discuss issues together?

Do you explore alternative options to choose from?

Who participates in the actual decision making?

What matters do the children decide on their own?

In what areas are the children simply given orders?

2. How well do the children follow either their own decisions or suggestions, and orders given by parents?

Parents' opinions:

Children's opinions:

How well do the parents follow either their own decisions or directions given by external authority?

____

____

3. When a child disobeys or acts irresponsibly, how do the parents respond?

____

____

What is done to help the child act differently?

____

____

Do these things work?

____

____

4. In your family, who has taken the responsibility to learn about diabetes?

☐ Mother ☐ Grandparent
☐ Father ☐ Other ____________________
☐ Child

5. Does the family as a whole
follow a healthful lifestyle? __________
A moderate and balanced diet? __________
Regular physical activity? __________
Effective stress management? __________
Emotional stability? __________

6. What major challenges other than diabetes face you and your family?

____

____

____

Your answers may suggest areas where your family could strengthen its ability to cope with diabetes and other life challenges. Parents can use the results of this exercise to discuss possible changes, first between themselves and then with the whole family.

Choosing a Successful Program

The underlying approach of this book is respect for the capacity of the person with diabetes to make wise self-care choices. The best diabetes program is individualized, with as many choices as possible coming from the child. Your attitude is crucial: children are better able to follow programs when their parents support rather than threaten them.

As the parent of a child or teenager, you may wonder if these beliefs are fully applicable without risk to your child. Can a child of five or six make wise choices to handle precise techniques like insulin injections or home blood glucose testing? What will control the rebelliousness of your teen other than threats of future catastrophes if he or she doesn't shape up?

Many parents and youths have demonstrated this approach by sharing responsibility fully, discussing decisions together, and gradually passing responsibility on to the growing child. Children as young as five have learned to use meters accurately to test blood sugar levels and to give their own insulin. Children in the pre-teen age range (and many even younger) are using insulin pumps successfully.

Rebelliousness may be an inevitable part of the teen years, but there is little evidence that coercion and threats are an effective way of handling it. Instead, give a teenager positive reinforcement and opportunities to learn to make more responsible choices.

Which Program Will Work?

For all but the very young, your doctor/health care team, your child, and you must work together to find a program and level of control that will work for all parties. Often doctors advise moderating or adapting the intensive program because of the greater dangers of insulin reactions in childhood. Children are usually much more active and engage in their activities with such intensity that the onset of reactions may be difficult to notice. Often they wish not to appear different because of their diabetes, and they may want to hide their vulnerability. The level of awareness demanded by the intensive regimen might cause some children to become preoccupied with their illness and some parents to become obsessive about it.

On the other hand, with the right combination of child, parents, and doctor, many children have learned to manage diabetes very carefully and live full, exuberant lives. Today, there are many variations of insulin regimens that provide great flexibility and can minimize the risk of reactions. The decision about the level of regimen a child is to learn to follow must be reached through thoughtful discussion between the whole family and the physician/health care team. The factors you will need to balance include:

- The long-term value of avoiding chronic high blood sugar levels.
- The need to avoid frequent insulin reactions.
- Your own and your child's feelings.
- Your child's age and learning skills.
- Your child's growth pattern and overall health (chronically high blood sugar can slow growth and the onset of puberty).
- Your child's activity patterns, sports schedules, lifestyle, and other personal preferences.

Avoiding Complications

Diabetes carries with it the risk of secondary disorders that may develop later in life. No subject in parenting requires more sensitivity than these possible complications. Along with insulin reactions and diabetic coma, future complications constitute a major threat and source of fear for parents and children alike. When your child begins to be aware of diabetic complications, you will need to convey carefully the nature of the threat and tell your child what to do to reduce the risk. (Your child may come to you in distress after hearing of a relative or friend of the family who has diabetes and has developed serious complications.) Tell your child:

- Some people with diabetes develop a complication, but many do not. The authors of this book (after well over 120 years of diabetes altogether) all see clearly, have no kidney disease, and have only minor complications.
- People with diabetes can do many things to lessen their risk of developing complications.
- Treatment for diabetic complications is improving; in many cases, treatment enables the person with diabetes to avoid disabilities altogether.
- Everyone is at risk and has to learn to deal with the fears this produces. Life has threats, but we live well by remembering life's promises more than the threats.
- The answers to any questions he brings up. But don't flood him or her with too much information. Keep a balance between the facts and the emotional reassurance you offer.

You should not force information about complications on your child, and, above all, you should never use threats of dire consequences to encourage your child's self-care. Either practice is likely to build more anxiety than adherence. Carefully inspect any booklets or audiovisual presentations on complications before using them. Old educational materials often use frightening, worst-case photos and threatening language. Even current publications on complications are seldom written with sensitivity to the emotional needs of the reader.

Before discussing complications with your child, read Appendix 2, pages 234–235. Deal with your own feelings about these threats first, so you can be calm in helping your child.

Minimizing Power Struggles

Any parents and children may develop power struggles over the children's behavior. With diabetes, however, these conflicts can take on an extreme level of emotion when "not doing the right thing" appears to threaten the child's very survival. As the parent, you may feel anxious, frantic, and possibly angry when your child "forgets" insulin repeatedly or eats excessive amounts of sweets. If your anxiety causes you to try to force your child to follow a certain program, you may simply incite your child to rebel even more.

You can do several things to avoid turning a matter of such genuine concern into a full power struggle:

- Deal with your own feelings apart from the situation. Don't dump them on your child.
- Ask your child to help you understand what is happening and what changes are needed to handle the problem. Work with your child rather than giving commands.
- Look at your child's behavior in terms of what is happening in his or her life. Does having diabetes reward your child with attention? Allow him or her to escape obligations or responsibilities? Help express feelings he or she can't express directly? How can you help satisfy these needs directly?
- Are there barriers—knowledge or skill related, social, attitudinal, or environmental—that are impeding the desirable behaviors?
- Set goals together, with a clear understanding of how you will both know when they are met. If it fits your parenting style, set appropriate rewards and penalties.
- Work with the basic understanding that you have a problem to solve together, not that your child is the problem.

Finally, understand that in some matters of diabetes care programs there is room for a few little vacations. Sweets, for instance, are not poison to a person with diabetes; they are simply something to be eaten in moderation. Don't let your child think that the only time he or she can eat a dessert or piece of candy is during an insulin reaction. Teach yourself and your child how to enjoy a flexible meal plan.

You might try having diabetes yourself for a day. Test your blood several times a day, take injections of sterile water, stick to your meal plan, and follow an activity or exercise program. If you care to enter into your child's reality in this way, you will discover a new level of respect for what he or she must do each day. And your youngster will be delighted that you have taken this dramatic step to live as he does.

The empathy this experience provides is the foundation for good parenting. When your love for your child is sup-

The Kid Inside Ernie Says:

One dumb thing I had to get over when I was a kid was pretending not to have diabetes. For a long time, I ate whatever I wanted (usually when no one was looking). I even forgot shots and ended up in the hospital in a coma one time. I thought if I acted like I didn't have diabetes, it would just go away. But it didn't.

I think I would have been a lot happier if I had taken better care of myself. I don't mean being perfect! But I wish I had remembered my shots, done my tests regularly, and not eaten sweets so often. I guess I thought the doctor and my mom and dad were the ones I did these things for, and I resented them for that. Now I know you do those things for yourself, not for anybody else.

Sometimes having diabetes makes me feel sad or angry or afraid. Don't ever think you shouldn't have these feelings. They are a natural part of you, and there's no reason to pretend you don't have them. When I kept my feelings inside, I ended up doing things that were worse than saying, "I'm angry."

The Kid Inside Gary Says:

My doctor wanted me to meet another young person with diabetes while I was still in the hospital. (When I was a kid, you had to stay in the hospital for several days just to get regulated). I was embarrassed to meet this person. It was even worse because he was coming to the hospital just to see me. I don't remember his name, but he was just a little older than me and he seemed nice. I remember him telling me that taking insulin gets to be a habit, like brushing our teeth. It helped me to talk to someone else who had diabetes. It took away some of my fear. At the time, I didn't think it was that important to me. But it was. I still remember it! It made me realize that even the most difficult things can be learned and become part of our routine. As humans, we are much more adaptable than we can imagine.

In a way, diabetes really helped me grow up. I learned about taking responsibility. I learned how to talk about diabetes and even other things without being ashamed. I learned how to talk to the coaches at school and the dietitian in the school kitchen. I learned how to arrange my life so that diabetes didn't interfere too much. I learned how to go out with my friends and do what they did and still keep my diabetes under pretty good control.

ported by this sort of respect and understanding, you both find that you can live well with diabetes.

Just for Kids

You're really lucky to be a kid now. The doctors and nurses today know so much more about diabetes than when we were kids. They're good at helping you learn all the things you need to know about taking care of yourself. They've finally figured out that kids can do all kinds of complex things, like testing their own blood sugar. Children are a lot smarter than most grown-ups probably realize.

Having diabetes keeps us on our toes—more than most people. Some great entertainers, public figures, and athletes have diabetes. Bobby Clarke, Wade Wilson, Brett Michels, Halle Berry, Sugar Ray Robinson, and Catfish Hunter have diabetes, and it hasn't stopped them. It doesn't have to stop you. With diabetes or without, there is a world of things we can accomplish if we really want to.

Believe it or not, every grown-up has a child inside that remembers what it's like to be a kid. The authors of this book

The Kid Inside Cathy Says:

When I was little, they didn't even have blood sugar testing you could do at home. Blood tests are a lot better than testing your urine. They help you know if you have enough energy for playing hard without having reactions. But remember, those test numbers are just facts to help you. They don't say whether you're a good person or a bad person. They just tell what your blood sugar is, so you can figure out how to change your insulin, food, or exercise.

It's a little like being a scientist. If your blood sugar is higher or lower than you want it to be, you can usually figure out why. Maybe you ran extra hard today. Maybe your snack was bigger than usual. Maybe you've got a bad cold. Maybe you got angry at your brother. When you figure out the reason your blood sugars are off, you're not only a scientist, you're a detective, too!

My doctor first told me I had diabetes when I was in the hospital for a broken arm. A clown came to my room to cheer me up and give me a balloon. I said, "I just have a broken arm and diabetes. I'm not sick!" I went on feeling that way and never saw diabetes as a reason not to do anything. I did everything my friends did, except for eating a lot of sweet things.

I asked my mom if having diabetes would make me different from the other kids. She told me, "You'll be stronger and more in charge of your life. You'll learn how to take care of yourself and eat the right things. That will mean our whole family will benefit because we'll learn to take care of ourselves from you."

All Three of Us Say:

We know having diabetes is a problem sometimes, but we want you to remember that having diabetes doesn't mean you're sick. You just have to watch some things other kids don't ever have to think about. (Some people think that makes us smarter than other people.) But most of the things we are supposed to do are healthy for everybody. You'll be learning about diabetes for a long time, probably the rest of your life. We hope there will be a cure for you to learn about someday. Scientists are working on it now, but nobody's sure when they'll find it. Until they do, take good care of yourself so the cure will work for you.

asked the kids inside them to write about having diabetes when they were young. Cathy was 10, Gary was 12, and Ernie was 14 when their diabetes started.

If your parents seem to be babying you too much, show them this page.

Parents: Read This!

- My child is an essentially healthy person who happens to have a condition that needs special attention, not a sick child who must be protected.
- My child is capable of learning to handle all aspects of diabetes care over time, not someone who must remain dependent on me.
- My child will learn to take good care of diabetes by following my model of healthful behavior and by receiving positive rewards, not from threats of the consequences of diabetes.
- I will find the right balance between my responsibility as a parent and my child's growing responsibility for his or her own life, including the care of diabetes.
- When I feel I can't cope, I will get the help I need to go on living well and aiding my child to live well. I do not need to sacrifice my life to diabetes.

APPENDIX

1

Resources for Living Well

As you've learned, living well with diabetes is a process, a process that relies on how you respond to information from a number of sources, such as blood glucose tests, your physician, or others with diabetes. Here, we list a variety of resources that may be helpful to you or a family member.

Diabetes Identification

You should wear, at all times, a bracelet or necklace identifying you as having diabetes and giving a number to call for information in case of emergency. The following service provides attractive I.D. bracelets and necklaces and maintains 24-hour hotlines, where details of your diabetes care are available to medical personnel from anywhere in the world.

Medic Alert Foundation International
P.O. Box 1009
Turlock, CA 95381-1009
209-668-3331

209-669-2495 (fax)
800-432-5378

Web site: www.medicalert.org

Organizations and Sources of Information

American Diabetes Association
1701 N. Beauregard Street
Alexandria, VA 22311

703-549-1500
800-DIABETES (Diabetes Information and Action Line and customer service)
800-806-7801 (membership inquiries)
800-232-6733 (to order books)

Web sites: www.diabetes.org (for diabetes information)
http://store.diabetes.org (to shop for books)

The American Diabetes Association (ADA) supports research, education, and public awareness programs relating to both type 1 and type 2 diabetes. A membership fee of $28 a year provides monthly issues of *Diabetes Forecast*.

National Diabetes Information Clearinghouse
1 Information Way
Bethesda, MD 20892-3560

301-654-3327
301-907-8906 (fax)
800-860-8747

Web site: www.diabetes.niddk.nih.gov

The National Diabetes Information Clearinghouse (NDIC) works to increase knowledge and understanding about diabetes among patients, health professionals, and the public. It provides responses to inquiries and resources for patient education, including publications, professional and patient education programs, and an online database. Call or write to request NDIC's publications list. *Diabetes Dateline* is the organization's newsletter.

American Association of Diabetes Educators
100 W. Monroe Street, Suite 400
Chicago, IL 60603

800-832-6874 (to find diabetes educators in your area)

Web site: www.aadenet.org

The American Dietetic Association
120 South Riverside Plaza, Suite 2000
Chicago, IL 60606-6995

800-877-1600 (to find registered dietitians in your area)
800-366-1655 (Nutrition Information Line,
9–4 p.m. CST, M–F)

Web site: www.eatright.org

International Diabetes Federation
40 Washington Street
B-1050 Brussels, Belgium

Web site: www.idf.org

International Association for Medical Assistance for Travelers
417 Center Street
Lewiston, NY 14092

716-754-4883 (for a list of doctors in foreign countries who speak English)
519-836-3412 (fax)

Web site: www.iamat.org

International Diabetic Athletes Association
1647 W. Bethany Home Road #B
Phoenix, AZ 85015-2507

800-898-IDAA

E-mail: idaa@getnet.com

Diabetes Publications

Diabetes Forecast is the most complete magazine for people with diabetes. Published by the American Diabetes Association, it includes reports on new research, personal stories, practical tips on diabetes care, and articles for children. Membership is $28 per year. Reprints and special topic packages are available. Call 1-800-806-7801.

***Diabetes Health* (formerly *Diabetes Interview*)**
6 School Street, Suite 160
Fairfax, CA 94930-1650

800-488-8468

The American Diabetes Association publishes many helpful books. For a complete list, check the bookstore web site at http://store.diabetes.org. We especially recommend the following titles:

Complete Guide to Diabetes
Complete Guide to Carb Counting
The Month of Meals Meal Planning and Cookbook Series
101 Tips for Improving Your Blood Sugar
Small Steps, Big Rewards book and pedometer package

Walking Off Weight Workbook, Robert J. Sweetgall (Creative Walking, P.O. Box 50296, Clayton, MO 63105, 800-762-9255). This is a great workbook that shows you how to develop an easy walking program.

The Complete Book of Relaxation Techniques, Jenny Sutcliffe (People's Medical Society, 1994). Everything you need to know about how to relax.

Music to help you relax:

Passages, William Ackerman (Windham Hill Records)
Music for Airports or Plateaux of Mirrors, Brian Eno (ECM)
Spectrum Suite, Steve Halprin (SRI Records)

Online Diabetes Information

www.ndep.nih.gov
www.childrenwithdiabetes.com
www.diabetesmonitor.com
www.diabetes.com
www.caldiabetes.org

APPENDIX 2

Complications Simplified

Type	Cause	Early Warning Signs	Prevention	Treatment
Eye Problems (Retinopathy) 2 types:			Blood sugar level control. Yearly eye exam by an ophthalmologist. Weekly self-checks for warning signs. Report any vision changes right away. Self-care measures on page 203.	
background (develops after 5–20 years of diabetes)	High blood sugar damages eyes.	Detectable by an ophthalmologist. Vision in one or both eyes may be blurred.		Laser treatment (very effective)
proliferative (more serious, develops after 15 years of diabetes or sooner)		Detectable by an ophthalmologist. You may see flashing lights, floaters, or blurred vision.		

Kidney Problems (Nephropathy)	High blood sugar damages kidneys.	Detectable by urine and blood tests.	Blood sugar level control. Tests for protein in urine. Self-care measures on page 203.	High blood pressure medications. Diuretics. Dialysis. Kidney transplant.
Nerve Problems (Neuropathy) 2 types:	High blood sugar damages nerves.			
peripheral (nerves to arms, legs, and feet)		Numbness, tingling, itching, burning, decreased sense of touch, sores, all especially in feet and legs.	Blood sugar level control. Daily foot inspections. Treat all foot problems right away.	Limited to improving blood sugar control.
autonomic (nerves to body organs)		Impotence, difficulty urinating, bladder infection, stomach upset, dizziness.	Quit smoking. Self-care measures on page 203.	Implants, constriction rings, or medication for impotence. Symptomatic treatment of other problems.

APPENDIX 3

Some Type 2 Diabetes Medications

Class	Name	Brand Name	How It Works	Pros	Cons
Sulfonylureas	glipizide glyburide glimepiride	Glucotrol, XL Diabeta, Micronase, Glynase PresTab Amaryl	Stimulates the pancreas to secrete more insulin.	Work well in combination with biguanides. Good choice if you are normal- or underweight.	Can cause hypoglycemia and weight gain.
Biguanides	metformin metformin + glyburide (a sulfonylurea) glipizide/ metformin	Glucophage Glucovance Metaglip	Decreases liver glucose production and increases muscle glucose uptake.	Good choice if you have high overnight blood sugar levels or are overweight. Can lower cholesterol.	Can cause mild, temporary nausea and diarrhea. Not used in people with kidney or liver problems.

Alpha-Glucosidase Inhibitors	acarbose miglitol	Precose Glyset	Inhibits the ability of the gut to absorb carbohydrate.	Good for reducing after-meal blood sugar levels.	Excessive gas at higher doses.
Meglitinides	repaglinide nateglinide	Prandin Starlix	Stimulates the pancreas to secrete more insulin in response to a meal.	Good for reducing after-meal blood sugar levels.	Can't skip meals with this med.
Thiazolidinediones	rosiglitazone pioglitazone	Avandia Actos	Decreases liver glucose production and increases muscle glucose uptake.	Often used in combination with other meds.	Not used in people with heart or liver problems. Must monitor liver function if using.

For additions to this list, as well as a complete list of all insulins available, see the January issue of the ADA magazine *Diabetes Forecast.* Every January the magazine's *Resource Guide* offers a clear and comprehensive update of available diabetes tools. Call 800-806-7801 for assistance.

Index

About the American Diabetes Association

The American Diabetes Association is the nation's leading voluntary health organization supporting diabetes research, information, and advocacy. Its mission is to prevent and cure diabetes and to improve the lives of all people affected by diabetes. The American Diabetes Association is the leading publisher of comprehensive diabetes information. Its huge library of practical and authoritative books for people with diabetes covers every aspect of self-care—cooking and nutrition, fitness, weight control, medications, complications, emotional issues, and general self-care.

To order American Diabetes Association books: Call 1-800-232-6733. Or log on to http://store.diabetes.org

To join the American Diabetes Association: Call 1-800-806-7801. www.diabetes.org/membership

For more information about diabetes or ADA programs and services: Call 1-800-342-2383. E-mail: Customerservice@diabetes.org or log on to www.diabetes.org

To locate an ADA/NCQA Recognized Provider of quality diabetes care in your area: www.ncqa.org/dprp/

To find an ADA Recognized Education Program in your area: Call 1-888-232-0822. www.diabetes.org/recognition/education.asp

To join the fight to increase funding for diabetes research, end discrimination, and improve insurance coverage: Call 1-800-342-2383. www.diabetes.org/advocacy

To find out how you can get involved with the programs in your community: Call 1-800-342-2383. See below for program Web addresses.

- *American Diabetes Month:* Educational activities aimed at those diagnosed with diabetes—month of November. www.diabetes.org/ADM
- *American Diabetes Alert:* Annual public awareness campaign to find the undiagnosed—held the fourth Tuesday in March. www.diabetes.org/alert
- *The Diabetes Assistance & Resources Program (DAR):* diabetes awareness program targeted to the Latino community. www.diabetes.org/DAR
- *African American Program:* diabetes awareness program targeted to the African American community. www.diabetes.org/africanamerican
- *Awakening the Spirit: Pathways to Diabetes Prevention & Control:* diabetes awareness program targeted to the Native American community. www.diabetes.org/awakening

To find out about an important research project regarding type 2 diabetes: www.diabetes.org/ada/research.asp

To obtain information on making a planned gift or charitable bequest: Call 1-888-700-7029. www.diabetes.org/ada/plan.asp

To make a donation or memorial contribution: Call 1-800-342-2383. www.diabetes.org/ada/cont.asp